Victoria

Bath & Beauty

THE FINE ART OF PAMPERING ONESELF

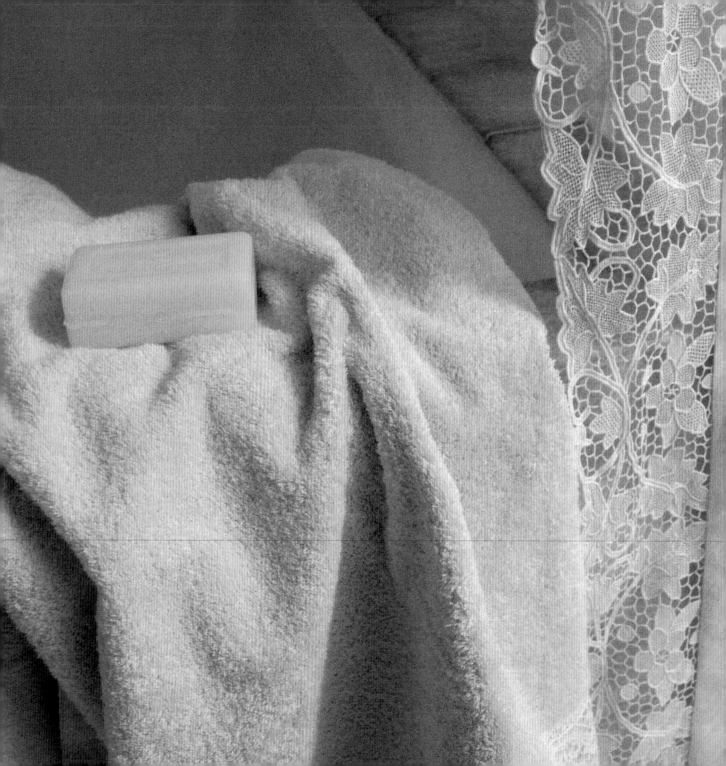

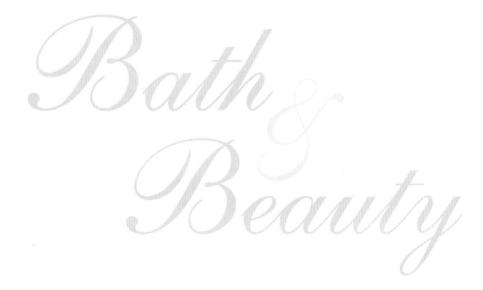

Victoria

Bath & Beauty

THE FINE ART OF PAMPERING ONESELF

Text by LESLIE GEORGE
Foreword by NANCY LINDEMEYER

HEARST BOOKS · NEW YORK

It is the policy of William Morrow and Company, Inc., and its
imprints and affiliates, recognizing the importance of preserving
what has been written, to print the books we publish on
acid-free paper, and we exert our best efforts to that end.

Library of Congress Cataloging-in-Publication Data
Victoria bath & beauty: the fine art of pampering oneself /
    by the editors of Victoria.
            p. cm.
        ISBN 0-688-16299-1
        1. Baths. 2. Beauty, Personal. 3. Bathing accessories.
    I. Victoria (New York, N.Y.)
    RA780.V53 1998
    646.7'1 — dc21   98-22767
                                                    CIP

Printed in Italy
Text set in Deepdene

First Edition
10 9 8 7 6 5 4 3 2 1

For *Victoria*:
Nancy Lindemeyer, *Editor-in-Chief*
Susan Maher, *Art Director*
John Mack Carter, *President*, Hearst Magazine Enterprises

www.williammorrow.com

Art Director: Tomek Lamprecht
Designer: Gretchen Mergenthaler
Editor: Carrie Chase

Produced by Smallwood & Stewart, Inc., New York City

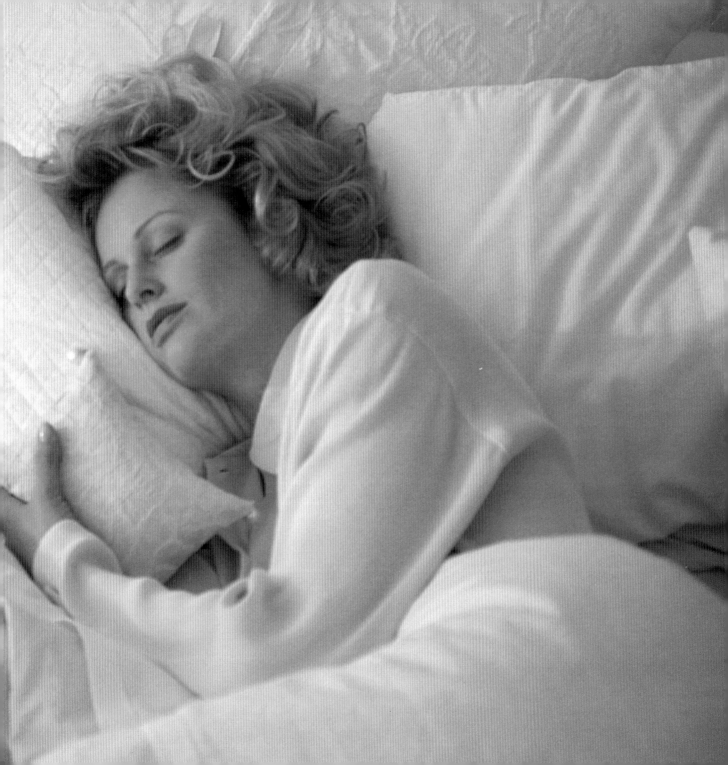

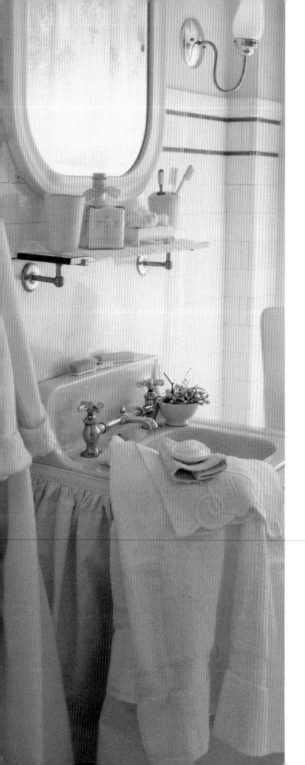

Contents

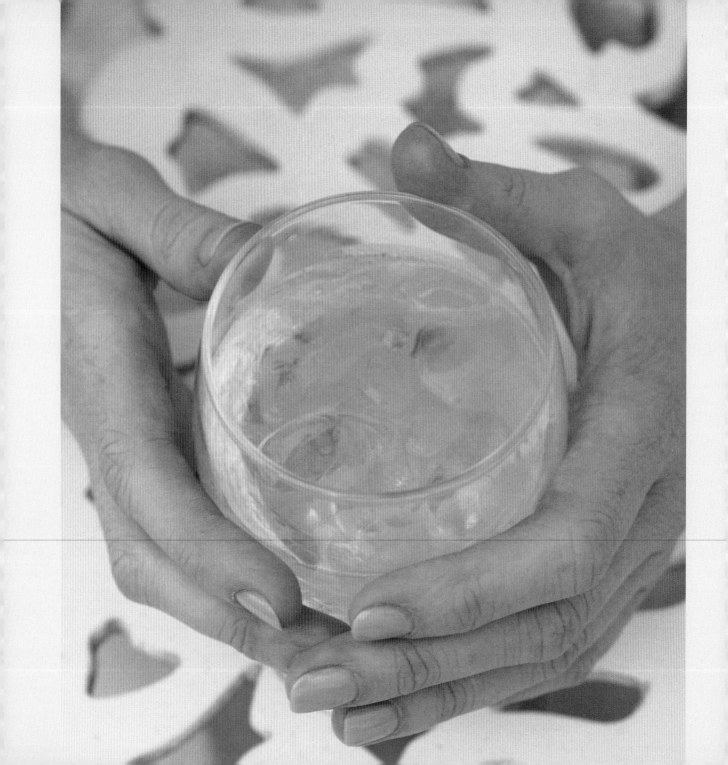

FOREWORD

One of my first apartments at the peak of a wonderful, old tree-shaded house had the perfect bathroom. I did have to dodge the angles of the roof, but it was worth it when I stepped into the claw-footed tub set next to a floor-to-ceiling window, three stories closer to heaven. From a nearby store I bought stacks of towels, and I filled a big glass bowl with bars of white soap. Oh, how I looked forward to the beauty rituals I entertained in this cozy place. The lesson I learned has stayed with me since—that a lovely bath both intimate and inviting is a grace we can't afford to do without. Wherever I have lived, I need those touches that make the bathroom just mine. My toothbrush in a hand-painted cup; scented soaps fit for a queen at my very humble fingertips. And when I had the chance the create a bath bliss of my own, I put in "miles" of drawers so I could squirrel away all my cosmetics.

Every woman dreams of a beautiful bath—and in this book we have filled beautifully illustrated pages with enchanting ways to make these dreams realities. When we step into a rejuvenating shower, stress vanishes. When our bathtub is filled nearly to the brim and we light a scented candle nearby, we have an invitation to a sublime hour. Use this book for making such pleasures happen every day.

— Nancy Lindemeyer, Editor in Chief

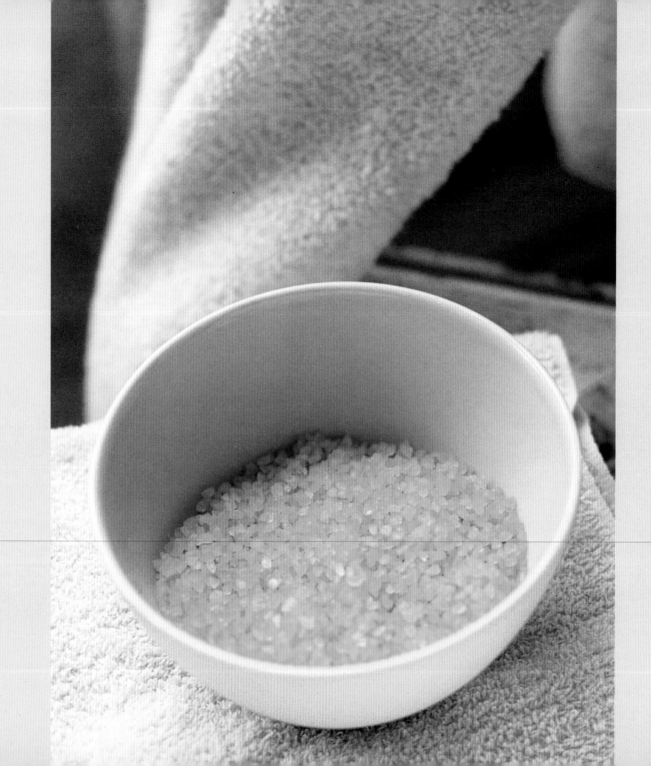

INTRODUCTION

The art of taking care of yourself is a most private need and reflects on your most public face. Self-care can mean many things in an ordinary week—searching at the cosmetics counter for the perfect lipstick, stealing a moment of relaxation in the tub, cutting herbs from the garden for a facial steam, meditating for five minutes in the morning, or riding your bicycle to work.

True beauty reflects balancing the needs of your skin and body, paying attention to your health and feelings. In this book, Victoria examines the many ways this is done, from taking a walk in nature to finding comfort and fresh flowers in the room that holds so many of our pampered memories and beauty secrets—the bathroom.

As the seasons pass, our beauty needs change, and so this book examines the elements of beauty in the context of a year. In these pages you'll find a guide to creating an at-home spa experience, and learn how to adapt your beauty routine for spring, summer, autumn, winter. You'll see exquisite details of special bathrooms, and discover the basics of skin care and the best tools for makeup application. You'll find new ways to appreciate each season, and your ideas about beauty may expand, as may your capacity to appreciate and treat yourself well.

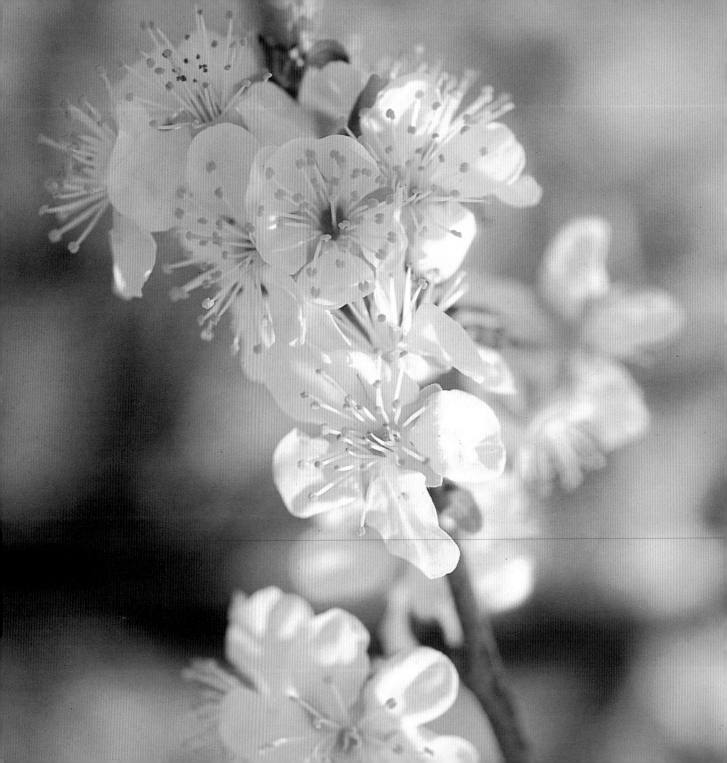

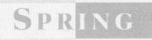

SPRING

Beauty blooms

Beauty blooms

alk outside when you are beckoned by the scent of earth, a sea of grass, the tender new leaves, the mood-elevating afternoon light. It is spring, a time to begin work in the garden and to move forward with the knowledge of the changes winter's quiet evenings have sown in your soul. It is a time to renew a vow to source your life from beauty. Think of the beauty of nature, and think of your own. As April showers—welcomed by Victorian women, who collected rainwater to soften their hair—give way to May flowers and refresh the world, refresh yourself, bringing new life to your skin, your hair, and your smile. To embrace spring, take leisurely strides, do not step faster than the beat of your heart. Nourish yourself with self-acceptance, with the scent of blossoms, and with the contents of a picnic basket that holds only your favorite foods. Look at the face of spring, for every season has its own, as familiar and surprising as a baby's waking from a nap. And consider your own face, with as much awe and respect.

> NOTHING CAN CURE THE SOUL BUT THE SENSES, JUST AS NOTHING CAN CURE THE SENSES BUT THE SOUL.
> —OSCAR WILDE

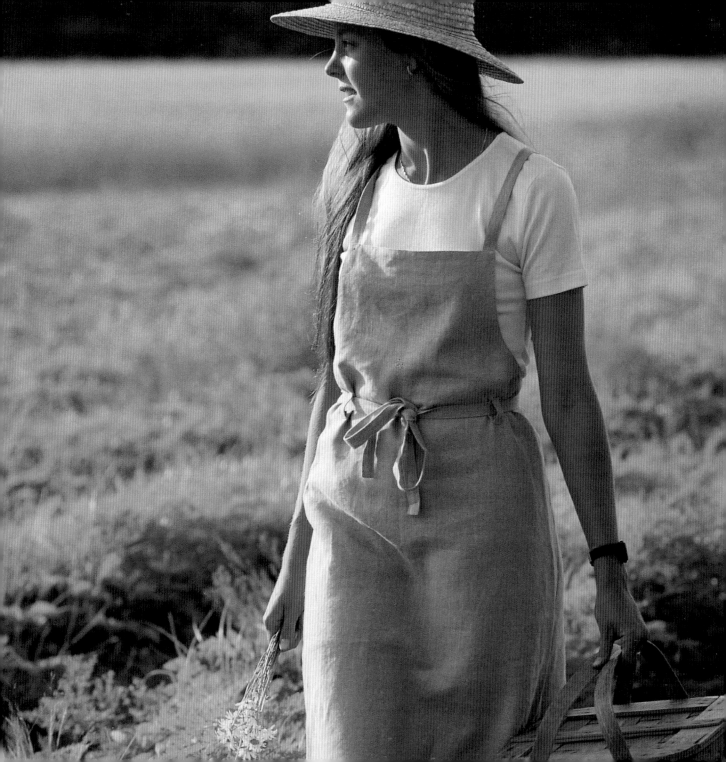

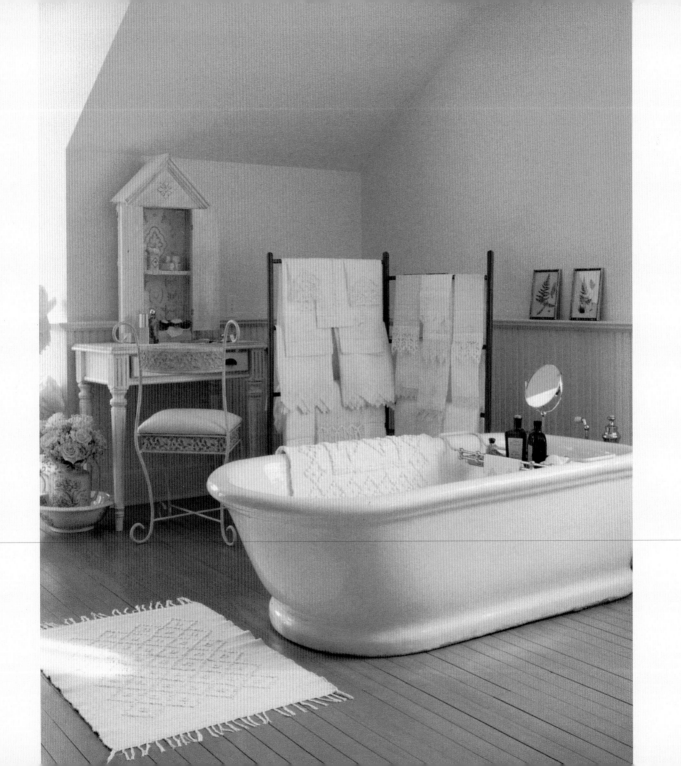

THE SANCTUARY

Close the door. Be still for a moment. Regard your private retreat. From the first visit in the morning until the last before bed, the bathroom is your inner sanctum. Your most unselfconscious moments are spent here, whether you are peeling off clothes, stepping into a bath, performing beauty rituals, or drying your face with a freshly laundered towel. The bathroom is the yin to the yang of spring fever. It is a place of temperance and calm.

In the Middle Ages, a sanctuary was a place of refuge and protection. Today, the bathroom is often the sanctuary of the home—a place made sacred by its quiet, because it may be the only room in which you are alone with your thoughts whenever you enter it. This

"INSIDE MYSELF IS A PLACE WHERE I LIVE ALL ALONG AND THAT'S WHERE YOU RENEW THE SPRINGS THAT NEVER DRY UP."
— PEARL BUCK

The time to meditate, contemplate, think, read— this is the promise of a yawning bathtub. Researchers have found that taking a hot bath an hour or so before bed can help you sleep. Late afternoon and early evening are also times when memory peaks. No mere indulgence, this chance to ruminate clearly.

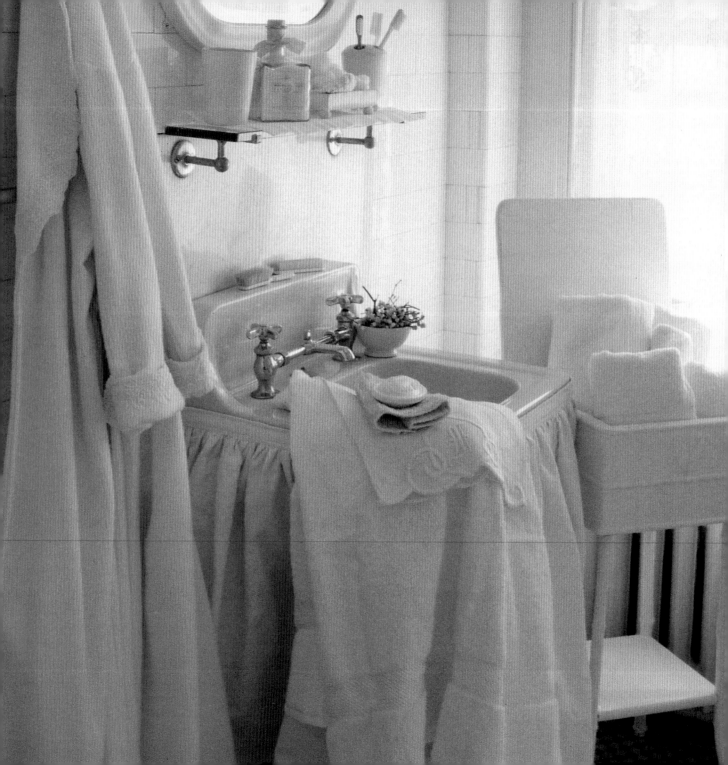

idea of the bathroom as a personal sanctuary—so essential to our modern lives—is a fairly new one. Until the turn of the century, a private bathroom was a privilege of the wealthy. Well-to-do Victorians created bathrooms both spacious and luxurious, others not so fortunate climbed up multiple flights of stairs with water from a public well. For centuries before

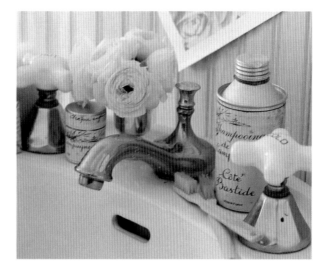

that, people visited communal baths, where they socialized as well as bathed. As technology developed, water mains were installed in major cities and hot running water came into the home, so that today we have the luxury of bathing in private. Be thankful for this, and consider your bathroom as your space of solitude, your chance to close the door for a few brief, stolen moments.

A toothbrush and a nail brush, a face cloth, scented soap, fluffy towels, and a long wrap-around robe are all that is needed for a fresh start. In the landscape of a white bathroom (opposite), morning light and dusk reverberate a certain comfort that also comes of being alone, of being home. A cluster of luxuries (above) around a sink's brass fixtures is a welcoming first sight.

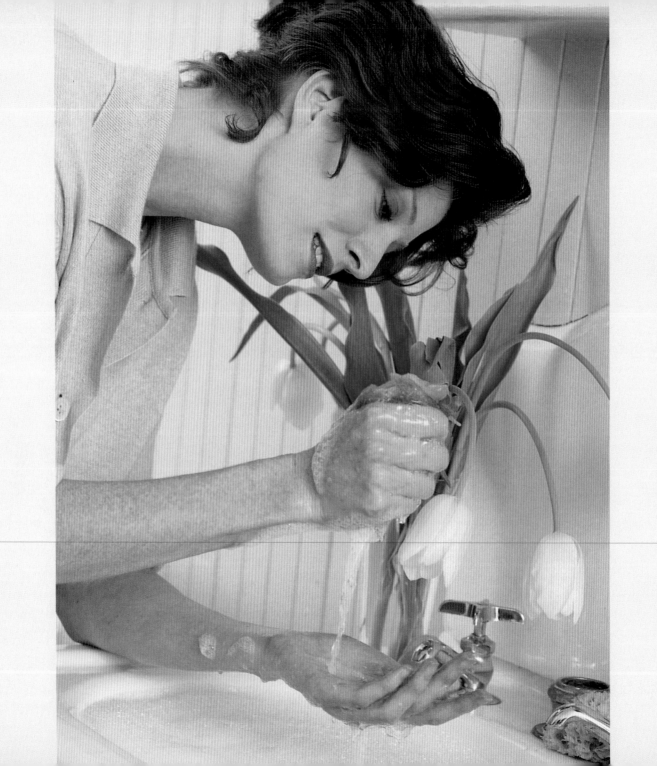

Because of its intimate nature, even the smallest decorative gesture has great impact in the bathroom. Victorians knew well how to integrate flowers into the home, appreciating that their joy could blossom even more fully outside of the garden. Spring flowers are without doubt the most romantic of all, and tiny bouquets play nonchalantly against the cool, hard surfaces of bathroom fittings. Appreciate how precious even a single stem, perhaps a raucous parrot tulip or a branch of azalea in bloom, can be.

In spring, bring out more delicate bath linens and cotton rugs. Add touches of your favorite things—antique lace towels or imported flower waters. Set out seasonal art—a pair of floral prints, a pressed flower collage, a wreath of fresh lavender created especially to air-dry in the room. You may want to consider greater changes: a fresh coat of green-apple paint, an antique clapboard vanity.

Think of the bathroom as the place to gather energy from within, to remember who you are and where spring cleaning really begins.

GLOWING SKIN

Exfoliation stimulates circulation and leaves skin glowing. The Japanese use a wood-handled, long-bristled tawashi brush; you can use a loofah or sea sponge, or simply a washcloth. Soften skin first with water, scrub in circular motions, moving outward, away from your heart. (For calluses on hands and heels use a pumice stone.) Be gentle, to avoid irritation, and don't scrub over blemishes or moles. Always rinse thoroughly. Then moisturize.

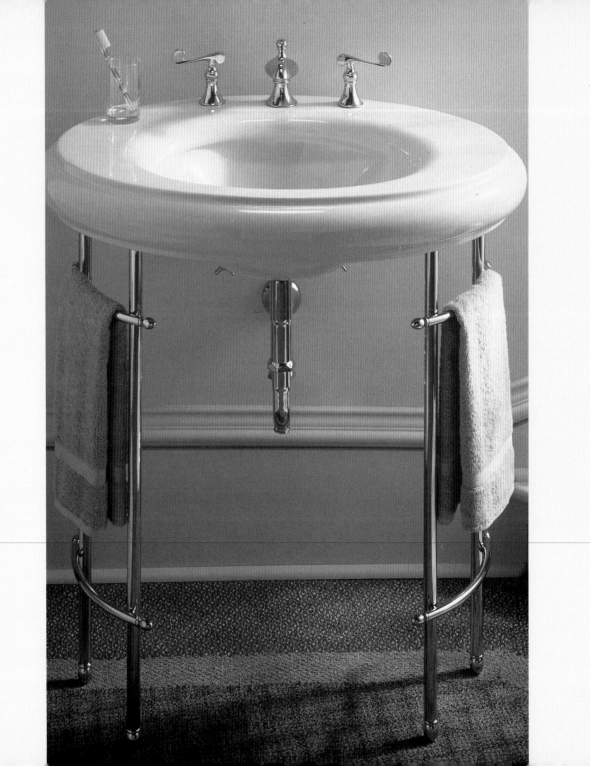

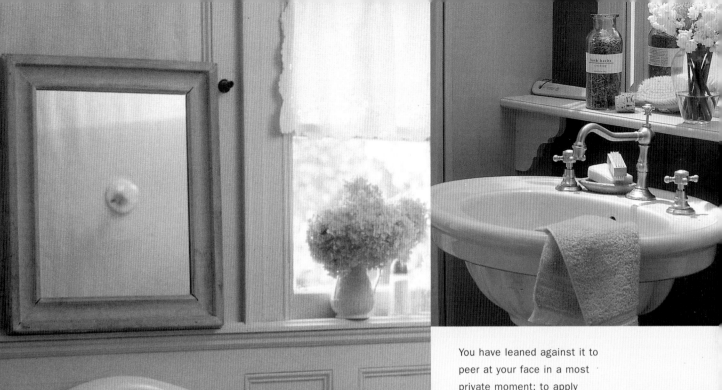

You have leaned against it to peer at your face in a most private moment; to apply mascara; to brush your teeth. This porcelain port of hand-washing and face-rinsing anchors your bathroom. Whether bare and upright or made to be fitted with a whimsical skirt, the bathroom sink can be more than a vessel of routine. You can make it a welcoming respite, a basin of pleasure, by lending to it a touch of your style, whether it be a modern commode (opposite), a turn-of-the-century basin (left), or a pedestal sink (top).

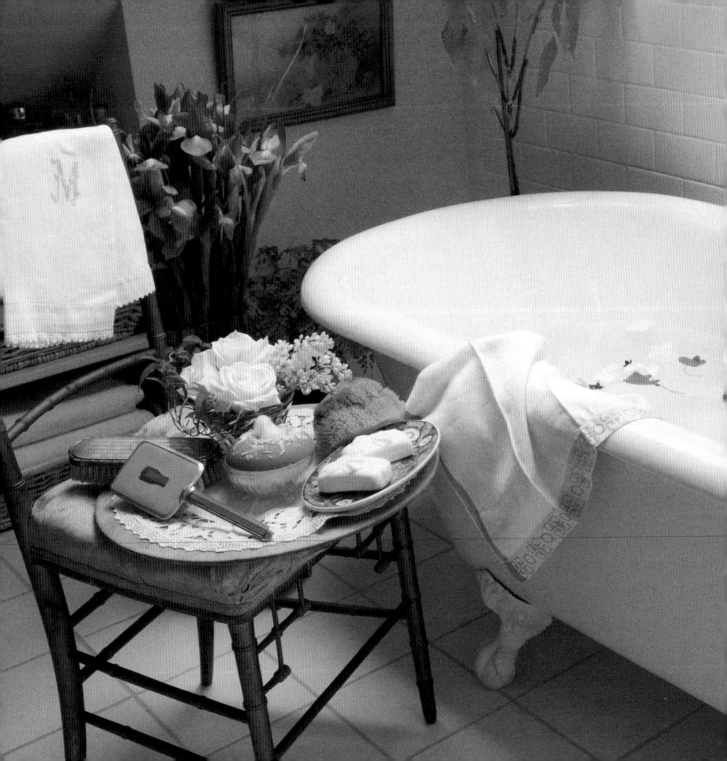

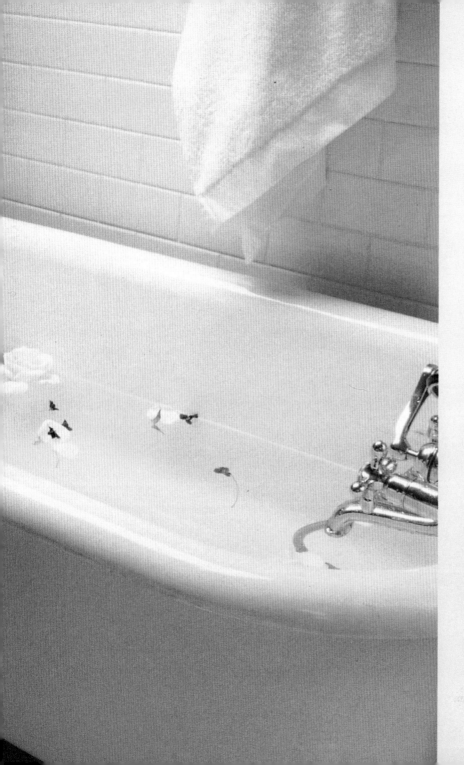

The ancient Greeks would consider it bad manners not to offer a travel-weary guest the use of a bath, during which oils would be rubbed on the body and scrubbed off. (Warm water, considered effeminate, would be reserved for women. Men had to settle with a splash of cold.) In this refuge, a handful of rose cuttings are added to a cup of bath salts. Drifting petals create lulling scented islands in this bath-time escape, an act of kindness a traveler, or home-dweller, will not soon forget.

INTO THE GARDEN

To know spring is to know nature, to be drawn to the scent of a leaf, to feel warmth on the neck from the sun, and to let tendrils of hair drift in the wind. Enjoying nature is a cornerstone of inner beauty. Experience the color green, a hue that lies somewhere between blue and yellow. The family of green fragrances include the aromas of juniper, hyacinth, and rosemary—all fresh, tangy, mind-expanding scents. Herbs and plants have been used throughout time to nourish and sustain the body. Their essences are distilled and used in the most effective cosmetic treatments. Cornflower is used in toners and astringents; eucalyptus in soaps, lotions, and perfumes; eyebright in eye lotions; honeysuckle in soaps; horsetails in shampoos; sage in skin purifiers; and St. John's wort in treatments for sun-damaged or chapped skin.

"TAKING JOY IN LIFE IS A WOMAN'S BEST COSMETIC."
— ROSALIND RUSSELL

Spring is the season of growth and development—for us as well as nature. To spring is to have energy, a tender bounce, to leap up or forward, and what better way to understand it than to observe a plant.

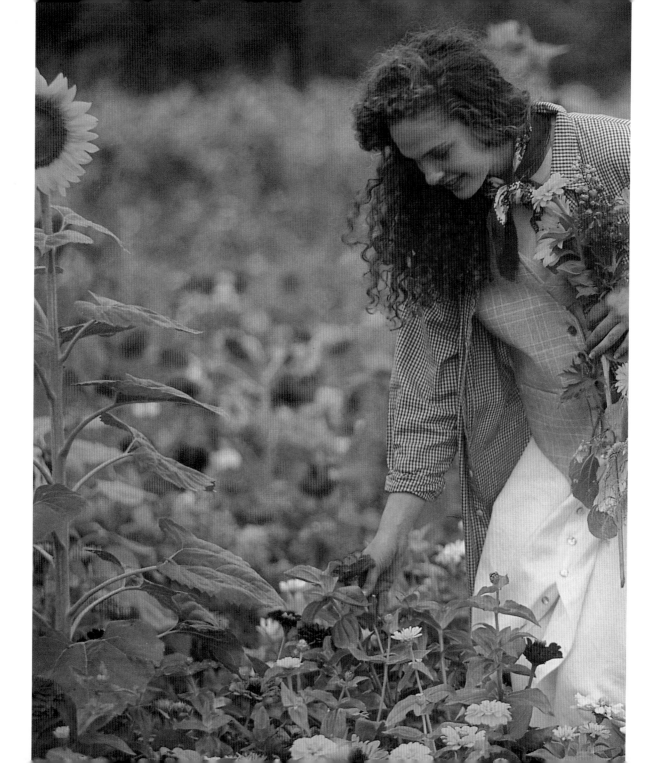

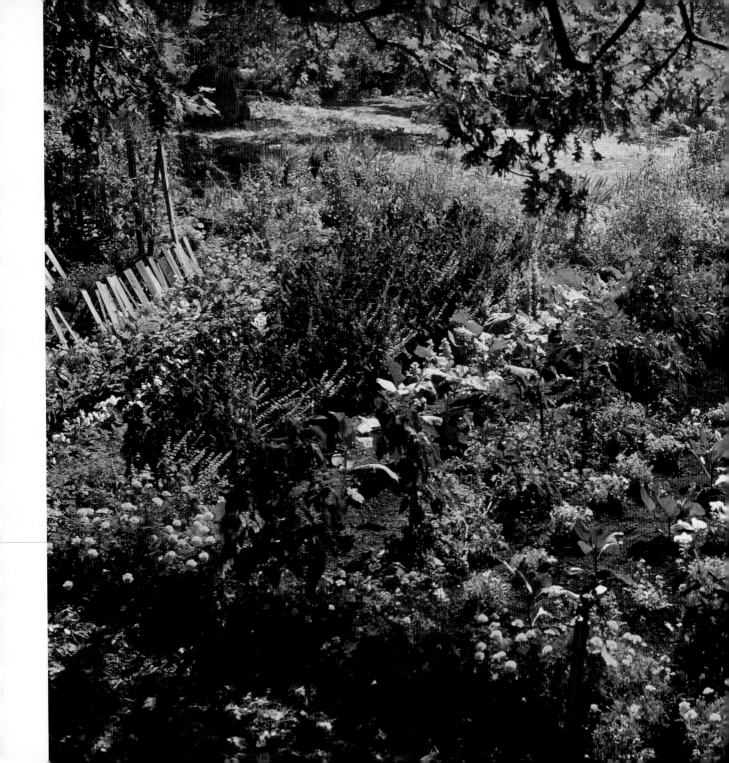

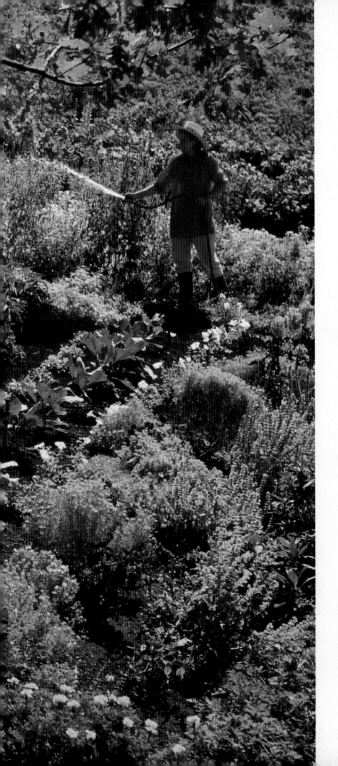

LEMON-TANGERINE HAND CREAM

3 tbs. avocado oil

2 tbs. almond oil

$2/3$ oz. (about 2 tbs.) beeswax, grated and packed

$1/3$ oz. (about 1 tbs.) cocoa butter, grated and packed

3 tbs. freshly squeezed lemon juice

1 tsp. honey

Essential Oils:

4 drops lemon

3 drops tangerine

1 drop neroli

Gently heat the first four ingredients in the top of a double boiler. In a separate pan, heat the lemon juice and dissolve the honey in it. Add the lemon juice mixture to the oils, stirring completely. Remove the pan from the heat and beat the mixture with a whisk until cool. Add the essential oils, blend, and transfer the cream to a couple of clean, small, wide-mouthed jars. Refrigerate until you are ready to use.

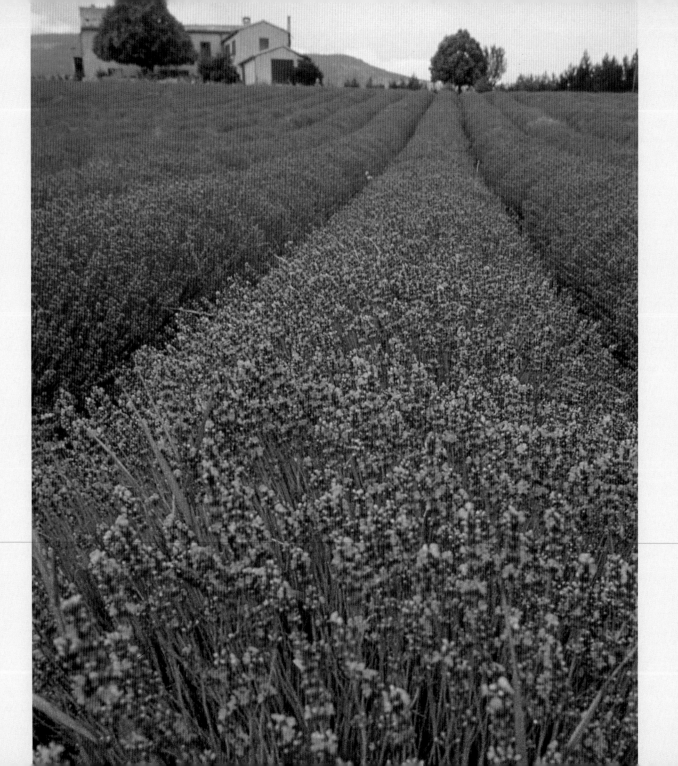

GIFT OF NATURE

Odors are processed through the right hemisphere of the brain, exactly where memories are stored—it is for this reason that the scents we are drawn to have so much to do with nostalgia. The latest perfumery innovation is called living-flower technology, which brings the wafting scent of spring to a bottle. Perfumers achieve these close-to-nature scents by placing glass jars over growing flowers or fruit to capture their live aromas, which are then computer-analyzed so they can be duplicated synthetically. But, of course, a walk in a fragrant field where the colors of spring make you squint is more therapeutic. The shock of forsythia, the allure of lilac are the colors and scents that stimulate birdsong and blood in the veins.

"SMELLS ARE SURER THAN SOUNDS AND SIGHTS TO MAKE HEARTSTRINGS CRACK." —RUDYARD KIPLING

Lavender, or Mediterranean mint, is a natural antiseptic and antibiotic that has a sedating effect on the mind. Aromatherapists use it as an antidepressant and detoxifier to promote healing and prevent scarring. No home should be without a bottle of lavender essential oil, which can be used directly on the skin without being diluted.

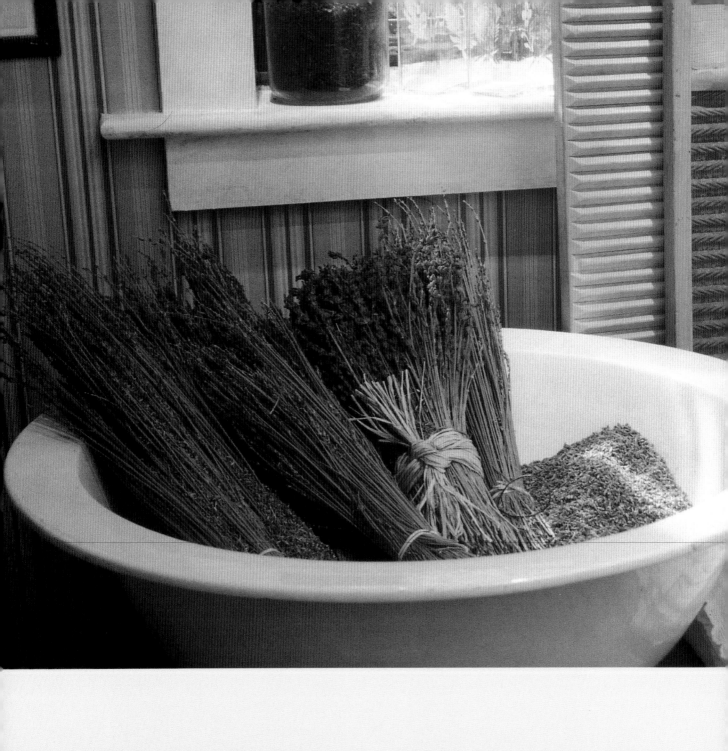

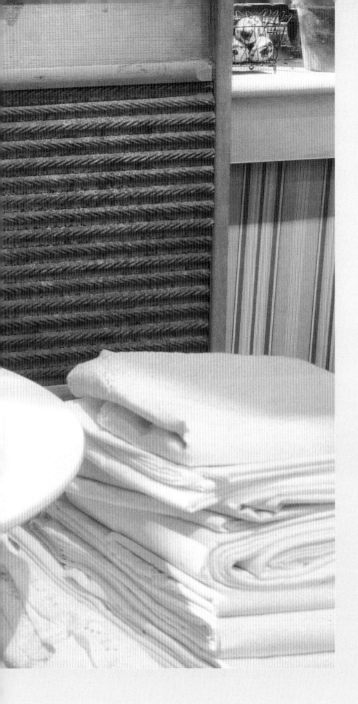

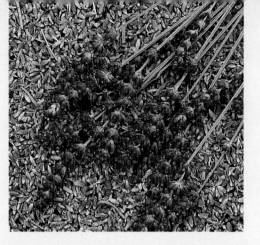

SKIN FRESHENER

This wonderfully effective tonic includes lavender, to help close pores, and rose, to soothe irritations.

2 to 3 cups lavender flowers
2 to 3 cups rose petals
Vodka or ethyl alcohol

Pack a glass jar with fresh flowers, cover the flowers with vodka or ethyl alcohol (available from a pharmacy), and shake daily for 7 to 10 days. Strain and add more fresh flowers, repeating the process until you've achieved the scent that pleases you. The final mix should be strained yet again, through a coffee filter or muslin cloth.

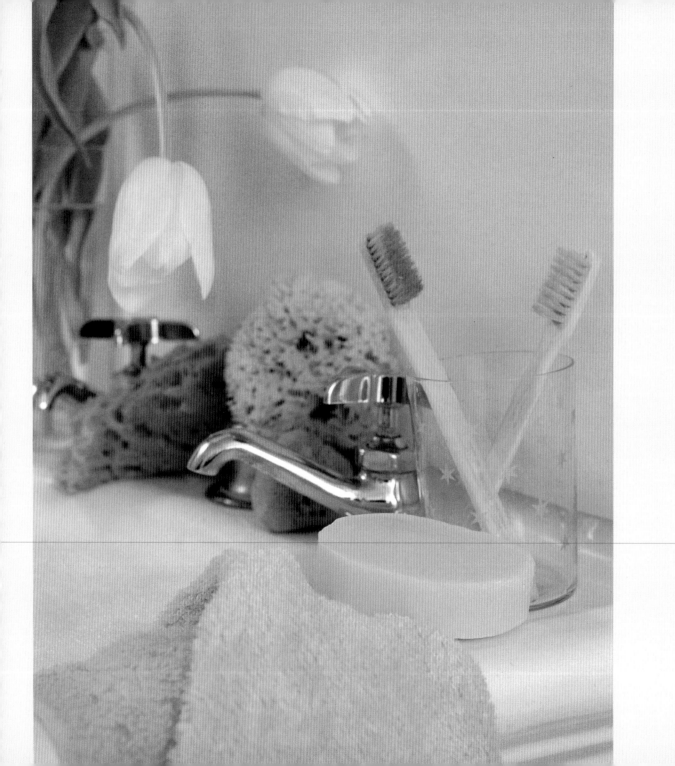

The French have an expression, *être bien dans sa peau*—to feel good in one's skin. Self-confidence, after all, is the root of all beauty. Then comes the skin. Fine, rough, freckled, dark, or light, skin—often ignored until a spot erupts on the face or until it is marked with experience—deserves your utmost attention and care. The heaviest organ of the body, if you could weigh such a thing, skin is built to keep toxins out of your precious insides, and to eliminate waste and regulate temperature through perspiration. Your skin also produces a natural protective oily substance called sebum—it is, in fact, the material that gives each of us our own individual scent.

Your skin loves water and moisture, and it's best to replenish skin with cream or lotion while it is still

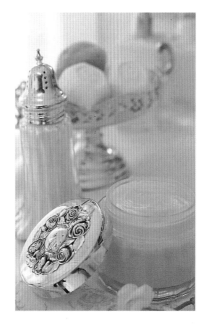

A refillable beveled jar with a silver-plated top and a curlicue-handled soap dish (right) show off imported tools of toilette, and make elegant additions to a bath. Sensuous in a more earthy way are a washcloth and natural sea sponges (opposite), whose job it is to clean.

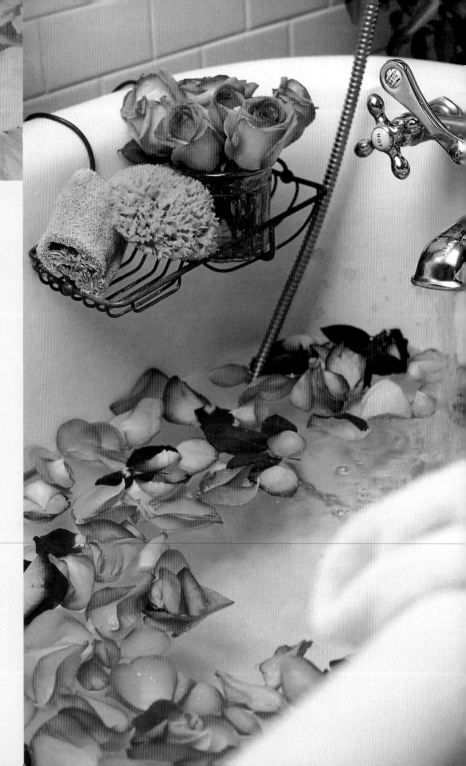

Sea sponges were once thought to be hardened sea foam; we now know that the porous mass of fibers is the internal skeleton of a marine animal. Its roughness removes dead skin cells and wakes up circulation, leaving a tingly trail of smoothed skin it its wake. Be sure to rinse a sea sponge well between uses as bacteria can build up. Another natural bath sponge is a loofah, which is the skeleton of a cucumber-like vegetable that grows on vines. If spring awakens the gardener in you, they are not difficult to grow. Plant seeds next to a fence in a sunny area; yellow flowers will appear on the plant first. Let the loofahs ripen on the vine, then soak in water and peel. Remove the seeds and dry in the sun. Save the seeds for next year's crop.

damp. Cleansing the skin, with bubbles or foam, oils or loofahs, showers or sponges, is a daily act of self-renewal—for the sense of touch is as vital as a drink of water.

This season that promises restoration and regeneration is a good time to look at your skin-care regimen and fine-tune it. Facial skin care is comprised of three steps: cleansing, toning, and moisturizing. The products you use depend on your skin's needs and should take your lifestyle into account. Before you begin, look at your skin. Decipher its specific needs for spot treatments—lines around the eyes, blemishes on the chin—then evaluate its overall appearance. Sometimes you may need an extra treatment on top of your daily routine. Oily skin, for example, may need a weekly pore-reducing masque; extra-dry skin may call for an occasional rich, nutrient-filled masque to replenish it. While you examine your skin, consider your day's activities. On days you don't wear makeup, you won't need as vigorous a cleanser. If you're planning to spend time outside, you'll need a sunscreen, even if the sun's rays may not seem too strong.

DAILY RITUAL

After a day in the sunny garden, cool and refresh your eyes. Chill a cucumber in the refrigerator, then peel and slice one end. Lie down in a dim, quiet place and place the cooled cucumber slices over your eyes. This will help to soothe irritated eyes and give your muscles a chance to rest, too.

To wash skin, choose a gentle cleanser that will remove dirt and grime but won't strip all the oils from your skin. From time to time, it is good to simply rinse with warm water.

- Spread the cleanser onto your skin and massage gently with fingertips or a washcloth for a minute to remove grime.

- Wipe off the cleanser with a clean cotton cloth, then rinse the face in warm water.

- There are several ways to exfoliate skin; do not, however, do it every day. With a sea sponge, massage onto your skin a cleanser that contains granules or one that contains alpha-hydroxy acids, which remove build-up by dissolving the glue that holds dead skin cells to the surface.

- Toners help remove soapy residue and close pores. Look for a water-based toner, as alcohol and other astringents can be drying to the skin, stimulating oil production.

- Always follow cleansing with a moisturizer good for your skin type. Usually a lightweight cream containing vitamin C or a vitamin A derivative is sufficient for day. At night, use a more therapeutic cleanser that rejuvenates skin as you sleep.

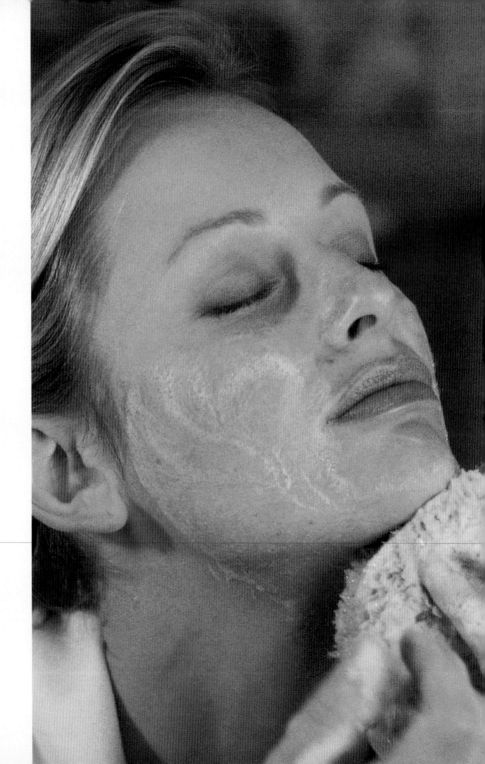

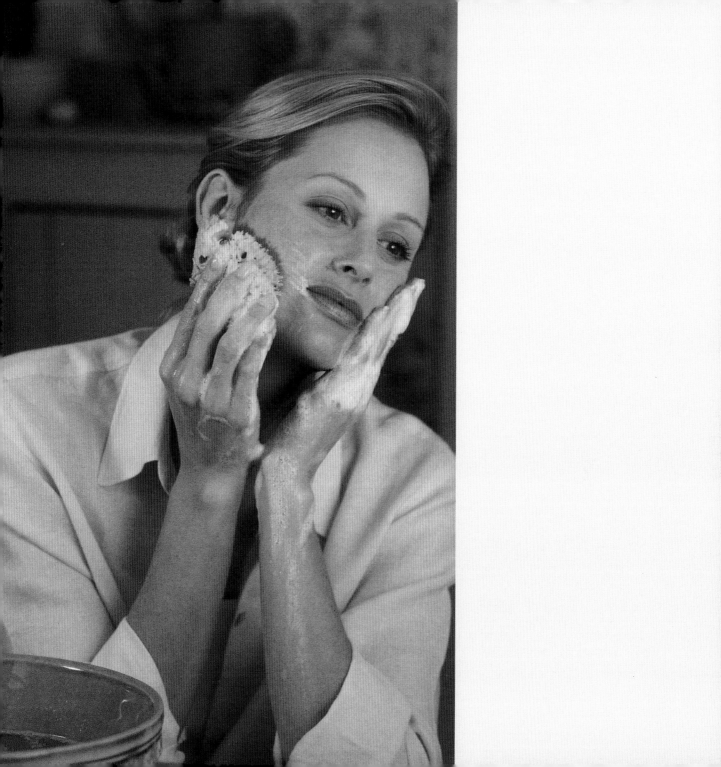

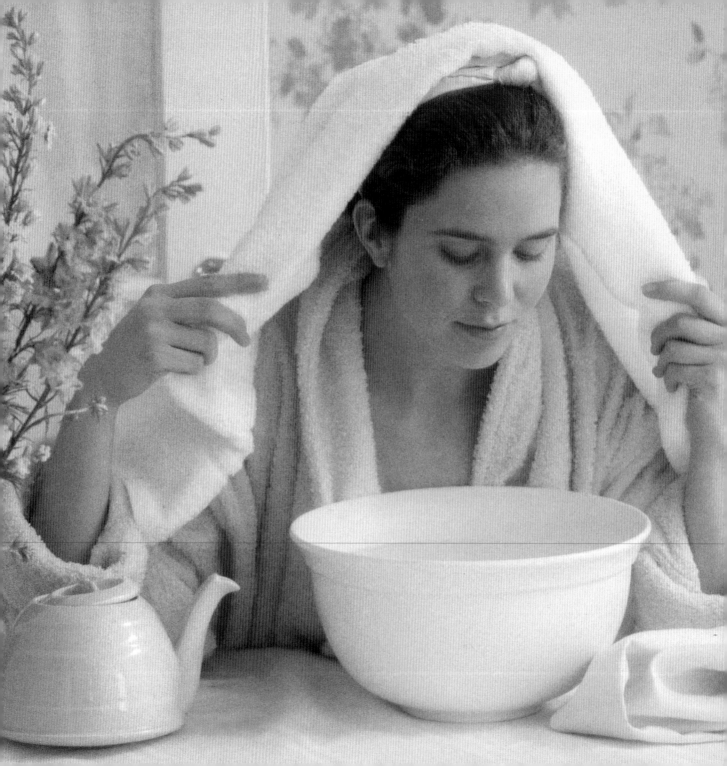

Spring
Rituals

Give your face a deep spring cleaning with a steam treatment. For optimal results, use this treatment, which helps to open pores, before a facial masque, up to twice a month. You can add a drop of essential oil for aromatherapeutic benefits—1 to 3 drops per pint of water; or a handful of herbs per pint of water for therapeutic results: chamomile for irritated skin; thyme, dried citrus peels, or oregano for oily skin; licorice for dry skin.

- Cleanse your face.
- Place herbs or oils into a bowl and add boiling water. For a "clean" water steam, add nothing to the bowl but the water.
- Cover your head with a towel and lean over the bowl; keep your eyes closed as some aromatic additions may irritate them. Steam face from 10 to 20 minutes.
- Air-dry the face. While skin is still damp, follow with a masque or moisturizer.

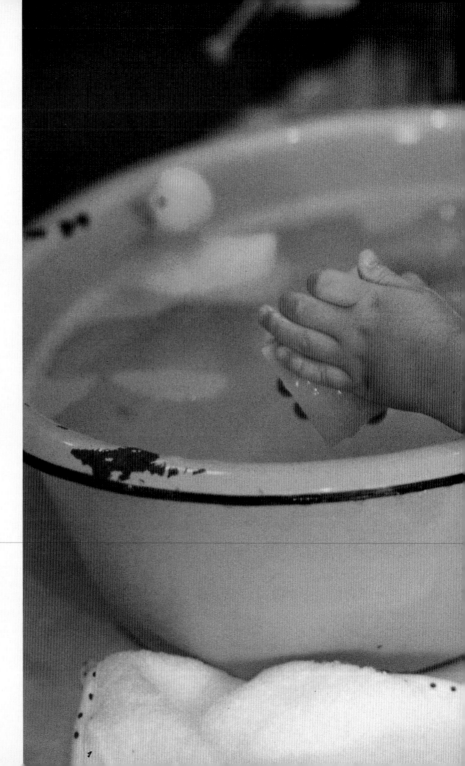

Wash your hands. It's the
first learned act of grooming,
empowering and playful. The
joys of it are the softness of
a slippery soap, the foam in
the basin, the fresh scent,
the feeling of clean. Every
baby knows the drill: Before
and after every meal, and
after every popsicle.

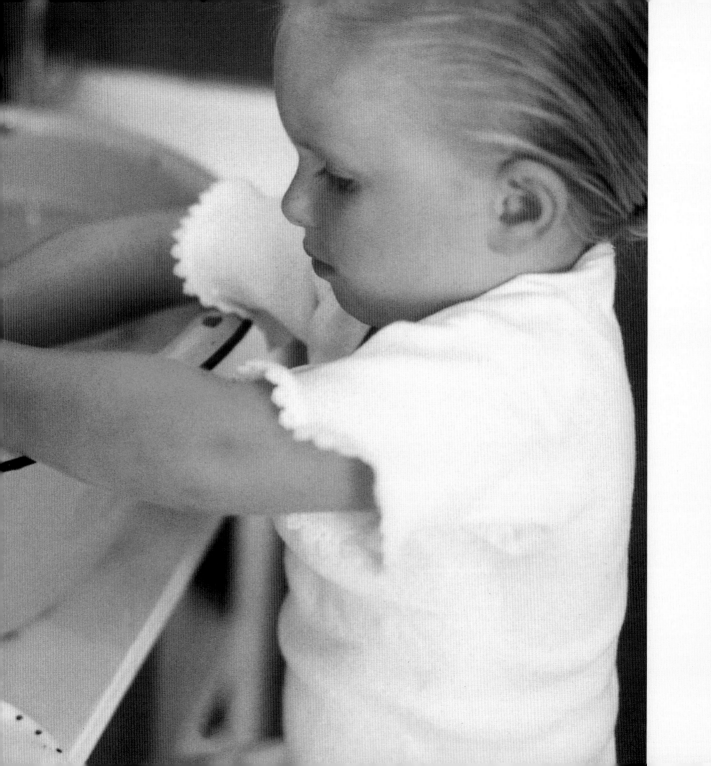

Pleasure of *Scent*

Jonquil Perfume

Narcissus flowers

Olive oil

Vodka

ADDITIVES:

1/2 teaspoons orange-flower water

**2 drops each:
essential oil of rose,
ylang-ylang,
jasmine**

3 drops lavender oil

1 drop clove oil

**1 drop styrax benzoin
(or substitute
Peru balsam)**

1 drop bitter almond oil

*P*ack a pint-sized glass jar tightly with narcissus flowers—any fragrant variety of daffodil, such as paper whites, may be used—and cover with olive oil. Place the jar in a sunny window for one or two days, then strain and discard the flowers. Add a fresh batch and repeat the process two or three more times, until the oil is scented as desired.

To each ½ cup of finished oil, add an equal amount of vodka. Shake the mixture daily for two to three weeks. At this point, the vodka will have "lifted" the flower scent from the oil and may be poured off. (Strain the vodka through muslin to remove any remaining oil.) Mix in the additives listed opposite to the finished vodka. Store in a glass jar or bottle.

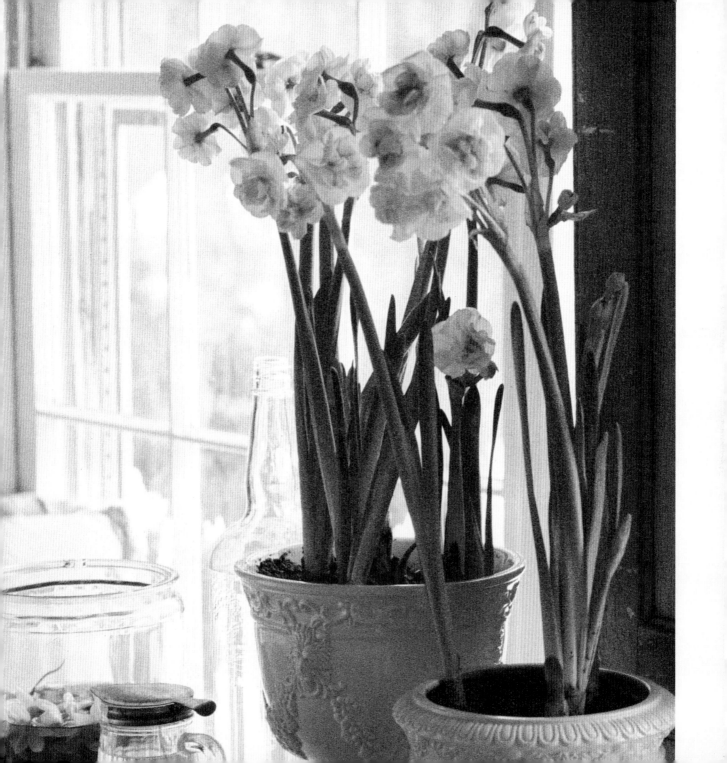

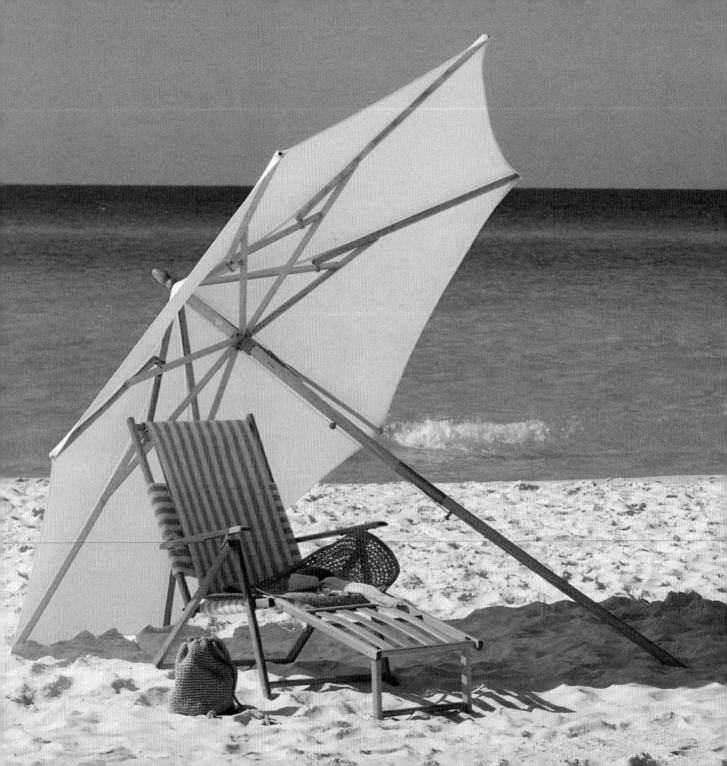

Sun & shade

Sun & shade

Somewhere between sunrise and sunset on a summer's day: straw hats, a hammock in the shade, towels on the line, red toenails, a secret garden, a bowl of berries, a beloved book, a campfire on the beach. These are scenes from the most unfettered of seasons, the season of having and spending time, the season of freedom. In summer we are our most exposed, even behind dark glasses. Our skin is naked to the world; our minds far from workday obligations. Weekend escapes, invigorating physical activity, stepping outside in the evening—these delights explain the light beaming from our eyes.

. . .THE SNIFF OF GREEN LEAVES AND DRY LEAVES, AND OF THE SHORE AND DARK COLORED SEA-ROCKS, AND OF HAY IN THE BARN.

—WALT WHITMAN

Summer beauty is easy. A walk on the beach exfoliates bare feet (for an easy foot massage, add sand to thick body cream and rub the mixture onto your soles). Humidity adds moisture to our skin and bounce to our hair. Working or playing outside increases the heart rate, boosts circulation, gives us space to breathe. Summer is also a time to find serenity in solitude, to remember the company of nature.

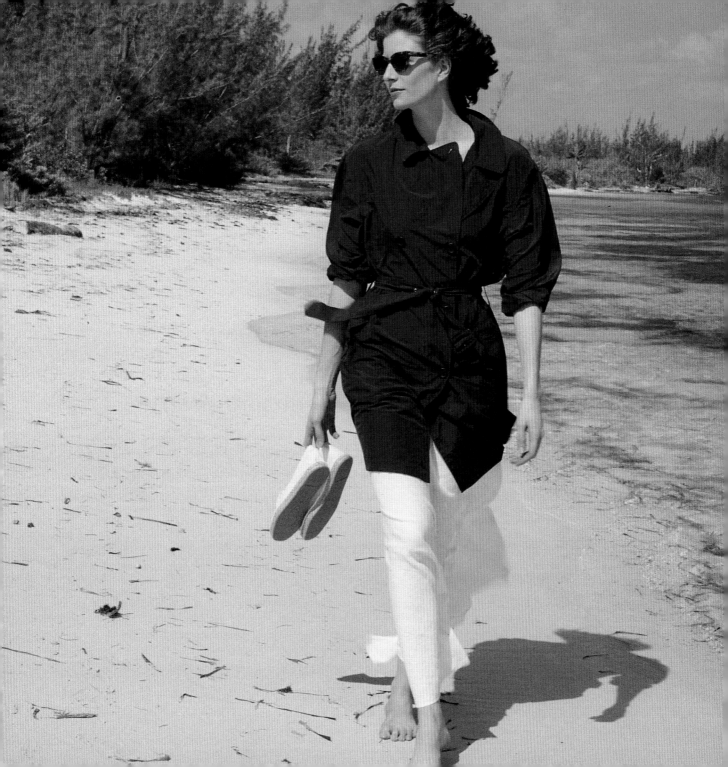

THE SPA

Originally used to describe a European site of flowing mineral springs, the spa has come to represent many different notions of health, beauty, and relaxation. From pricey bath products to a solitary retreat, the word is turned to when none other conjures a sense of revitalization, remarkable healing, and peace. The crucial element is water, without which there would be no life. The ancients knew well its healing powers; in our modern lives, we can endow the bathroom with all the accoutrements of the sanatorium "cures" with just a few flourishes—let light stream though a window, melt soothing sea-salts and bath gels in the tub, add atmospheric touches such as a scented candle.

The mood-enhancing effects of sunlight have been well-documented. At the same time, sunlight dictates our bodies' natural rhythms, telling us when we should

BATHE IN WATER
AND LIGHT,
A COMBINATION
SKINS AND MINDS LOVE

Use featherweight voile or chiffon gauze over a bathroom window to invite a summer breeze. More importantly, these fabrics welcome the light, providing privacy without darkening the room.

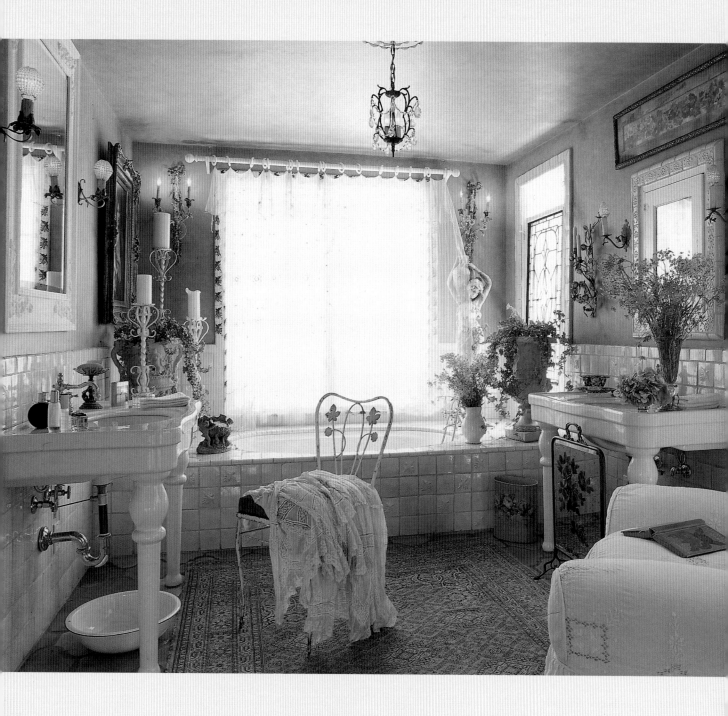

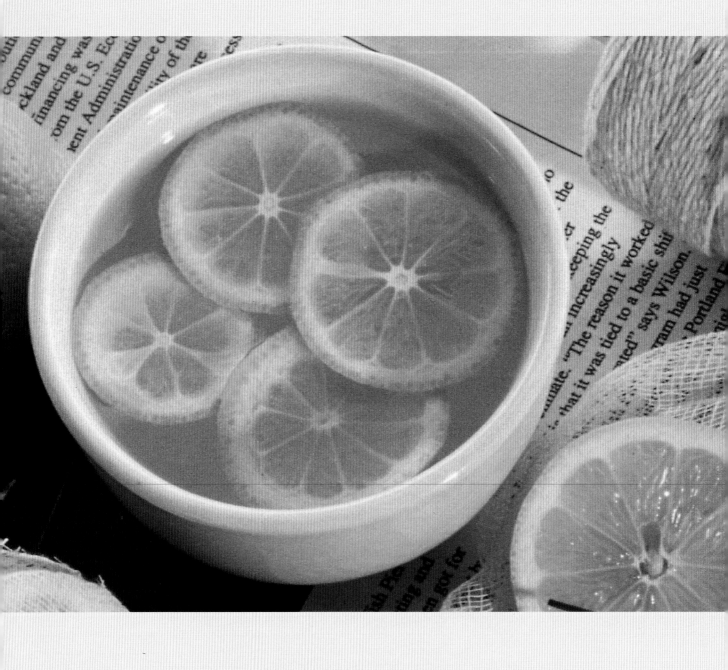

be active and when we should rest. Bathing in bright light helps to keep our bodies in optimum health. Those with a bathroom—or call it a lingering room—that has large windows are fortunate: they have the privilege of bathing in both water and light. Open up a skylight in a small space, and the effect is the same.

The water cycle—the continuous movement, powered by the sun, of water from the Earth's surface to its atmosphere and back again—is vital to life as we know it. Like Earth itself, our bodies are comprised of mostly water. And we need to replenish this liquid, as rain replenishes Earth. In ancient times, water had divine powers; Greek myth holds that Okeanos, the father of all springs and rivers, was conceived when Earth coupled with heaven. Ancient Greeks found knowledge and wisdom in water's caress; it is notable that we, too, can find spiritual renewal in life-sustaining water.

DRINK AT LEAST EIGHT GLASSES OF THE CLEAR FLUID A DAY TO KEEP THE BODY'S METABOLISM FUNCTIONING PROPERLY

The most refreshing summertime drink: chilled water with a slice of lemon. In aromatherapy, lemon is among the oils that induce positive moods, and it is said to enhance creativity, focus, and concentration. It can also become part of a beauty routine. Fresh lemon juice makes a simple toner for oily skin—add 2 teaspoons of juice to 1 pint of cold water, then splash on the face.

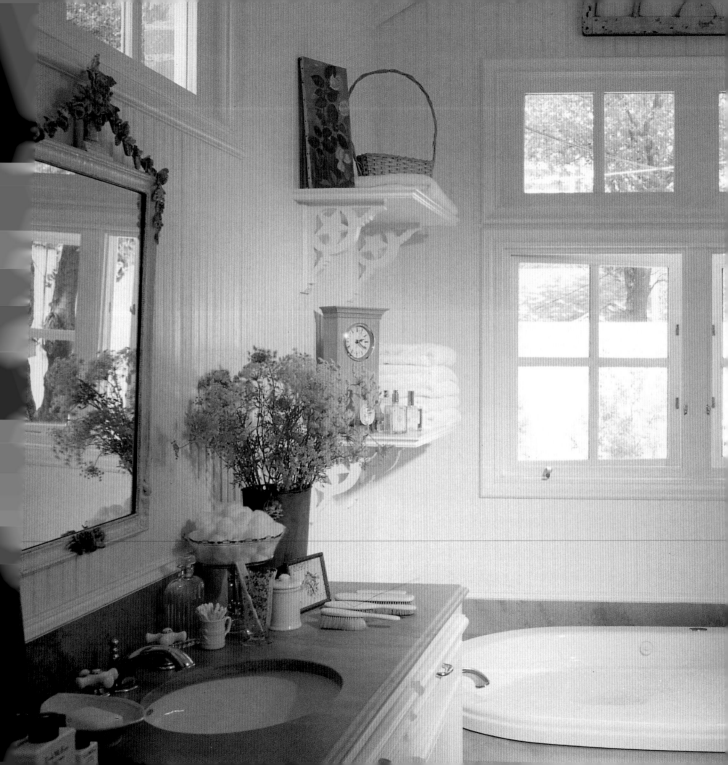

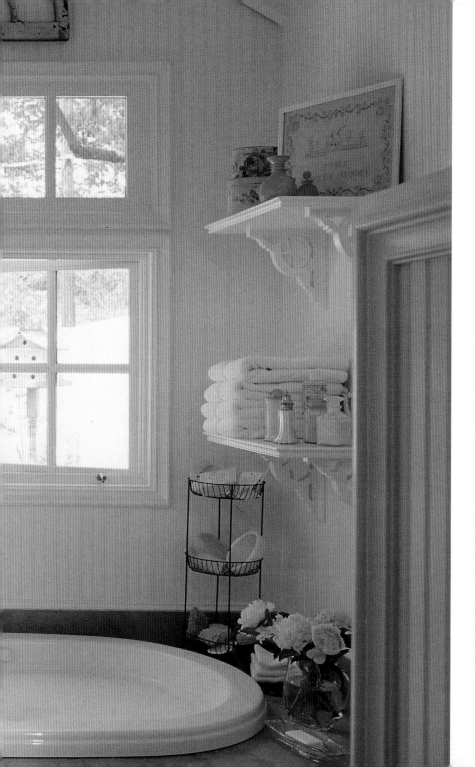

In this personal spa,
the bath is drawn under
a peaked roof, and white
painted-wood walls reflect
the mood of the day's
sun. As with any perfect
getaway—a tree house,
a bench by the rose
bushes—a room in one's
home can become a
place to renew energy.
This bathroom contains
the modern and refreshing
convenience of a whirlpool
tub as well as whimsical
touches of its owners: a
rose-topped, vintage mirror
over the sink, and bracketed
shelves that feature
celestial characters which
inhabit the night sky.

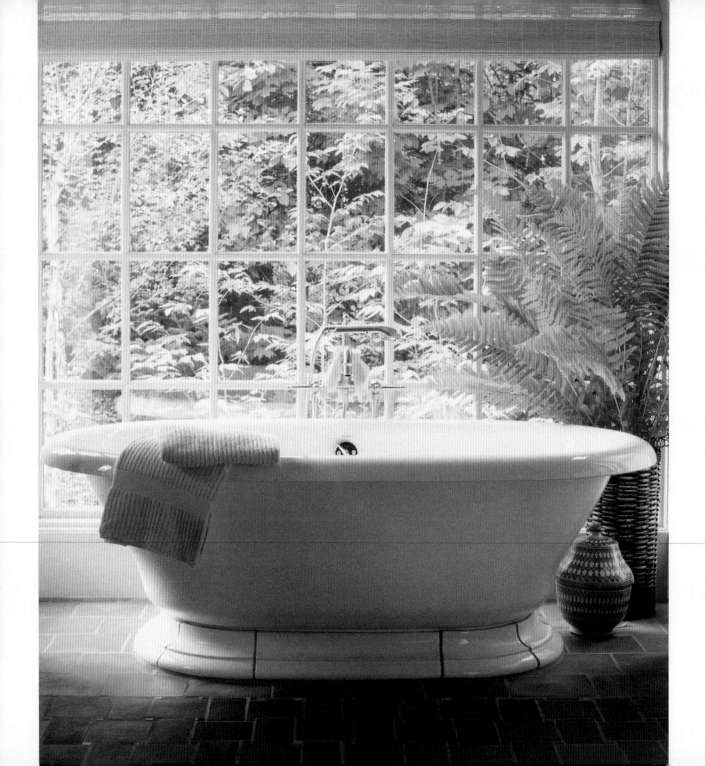

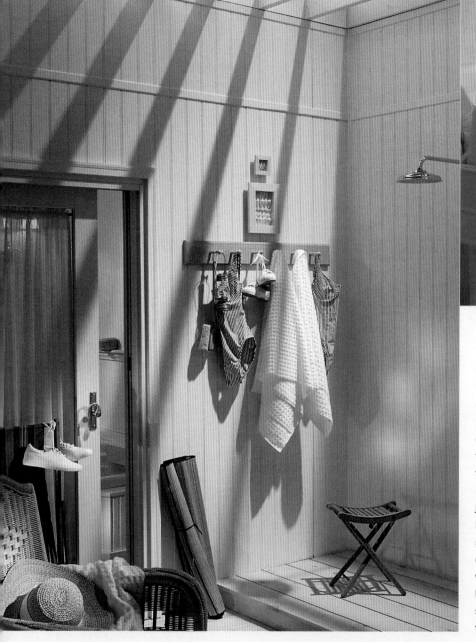

Bathing nearly out of doors—but protected from the elements—is an exquisite pleasure that can be enjoyed from the woods to the shore: An antique bathtub (opposite) sits beside panes of glass that frame, just barely, exuberant leaves of green. Enter this sun-dappled shower porch (left), and leave sand—and worries—behind. Keep at hand freshly laundered, sensuous towels (above) for the ultimate spa experience.

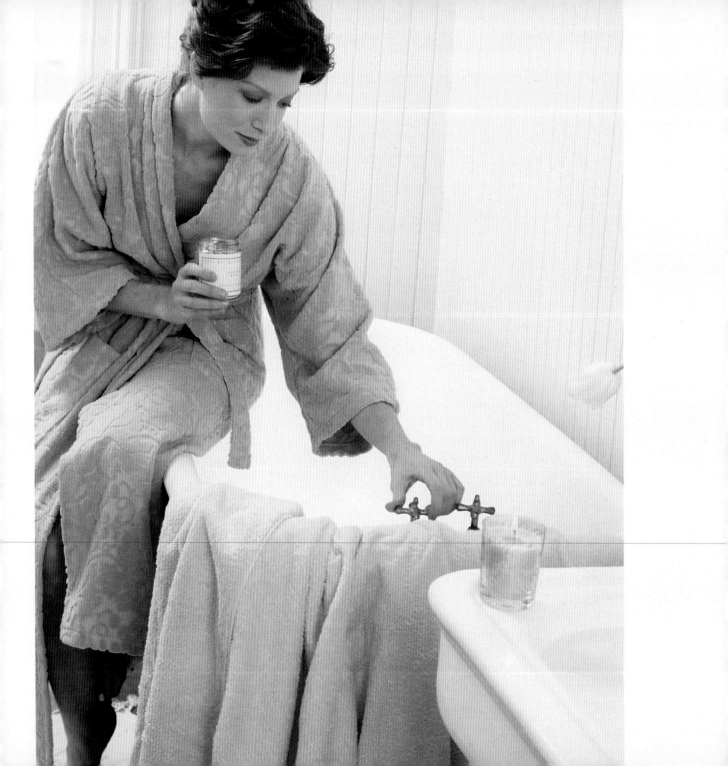

Early Romans were among the first to understand the truly therapeutic benefits of bathing. They made it a part of everyday life, recognizing the link between fresh water, hygiene, beauty, spirituality, and health. Their baths included steam rooms and saunas, cold pools and resting spaces, all with exquisite inlaid marble-and-mosaic walls under majestic, vaulted ceilings. Courtyards surrounded gardens of olive trees and cypresses, fragrant gardenia bushes, and trickling fountains, and offered thousands a sanctuary in which to socialize and meditate.

Like the ancient Romans, make your bath a multi-sensory experience. Let the water run as you sit in the tub and revel in its music. Use massage to stimulate skin and circulation and enhance relaxation. With your chin down, gently roll your neck left, then right. Repeat a few times, then massage both sides of the neck with your fingertips. Place your fingertips on your scalp and rub in circular motions; rub the soles of your feet and bring your hands up on your legs, massaging the muscles with upward strokes. Use the same motion on your palms and up your arms.

A WELL-LIT ROOM

If you can't bathe accompanied by the healing powers of sunlight, an illuminated candle will transform your bathroom into a cocoon-like atmosphere similar to that created at many spas. Remember that daylight is revered not only for its therapeutic effects, but is essential for correctly applying makeup and examining skin. If your mirror isn't near a window, invest in a chromalux light bulb. Light from this slightly tinted bulb blocks out yellow hues and illuminates your skin almost as if you were standing in sunlight.

OUT OF DOORS

Summer is the season to get back in touch with our physical bodies, to rejuvenate our muscles and our skin. We spend so much of our lives taking care of others; take time in the summer to answer the lure of the bird calls and take care of yourself. Venture outside, allow rejuvenation to spread throughout your body.

Regular exercise does more than produce a glow to your cheeks; it increases your life span and allows you to live with more vitality. Physical fitness prevents obesity, heart disease, hypertension, and diabetes. Inactivity produces the same effects in your body as aging, including muscle atrophy, decreased blood volume, and diminished muscle mass.

The American College of Sports Medicine recommends 20 to 60 minutes of continuous aerobic activity

"WE HAVE TO DECIDE FOR OURSELVES WHAT IS NOURISHING TO OUR SOULS AND DO THOSE THINGS OVER OTHERS."
— THOMAS MOORE

When the breeze is soft and the sun is warm, try to stay out of the car. Bike to the market, walk to pick up your children at school, row your boat instead of motoring it.

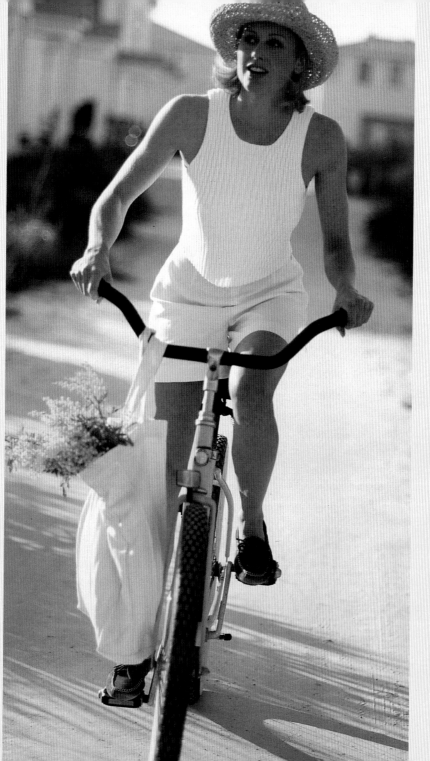

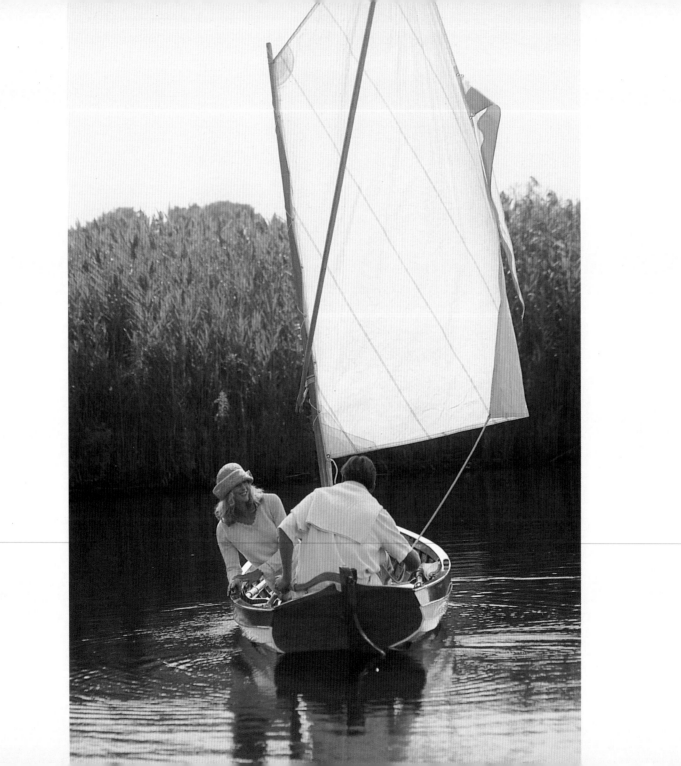

three or more times a week; weight training is recommended twice a week. Although most people know exercise is good for them, many of us don't get enough, so it's important to find an activity you enjoy—whether it is dancing, swimming, or hiking—and fit it into your weekly schedule. You don't need to go to a gym or hire a trainer; at a modest cost, you can buy a guide for an at-home conditioning program and small weights to strengthen muscles, increase bone mass, and help you lose weight without losing muscle. Remember, some muscle-building exercises, like sit-ups and push-ups, don't require any weights, just your desire to be fit.

Progressive muscle relaxation is a wonderful way to ease stress in your body and teach yourself the difference between tension and letting go. In a reclining position, breathe in and out three times. Starting at your feet and moving upwards, contract and relax each muscle group: feet, calves, thighs, stomach, buttocks, and on up. Hold for five seconds, then relax.

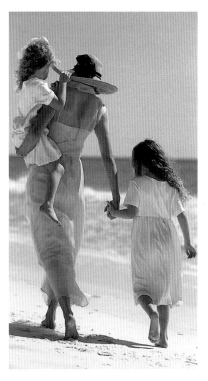

Whatever your exercise, in summer you're probably outside. As you tone and stretch your muscles, don't forget to protect your skin. Wide brim hats are essential for any time spent on the beach, and a sunscreen of at least SPF 15 is necessary to prevent burning and sun damage.

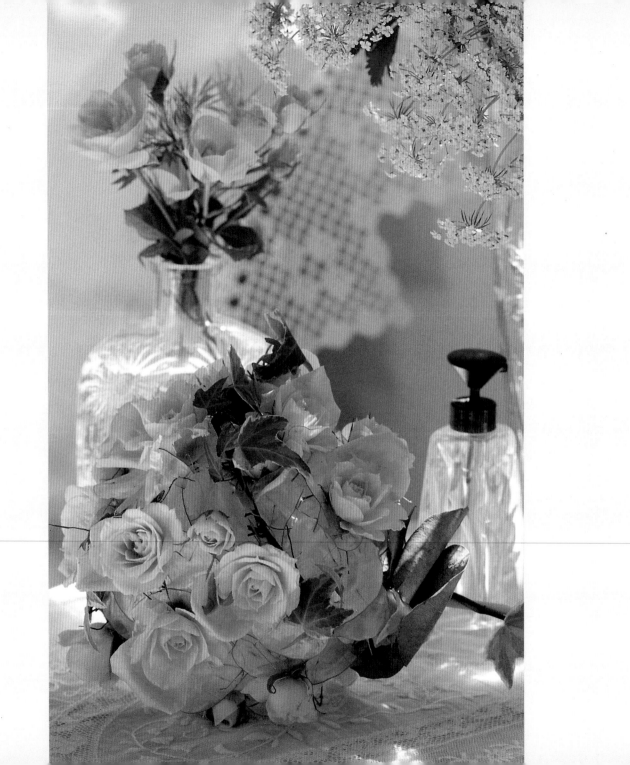

GIFT OF NATURE

With their profusions of color and intoxicating fragrances, roses are the flowers for which summers are remembered. A collection of modern roses—with names like Bewitched (pink), Spellbinder (ivory deepening to a blush pink), and Seashell (luminous peach, pink, and coral)—sounds more like a handful of makeup shades than an assortment of flowers. Antique roses have the most exquisite scent, and if you're fortunate enough to have some blooming in your garden, make your own rose water by steeping the petals in distilled water. Roses are naturally hydrating, which is one reason why they are so often included in beauty products; their ancient association with love and romance is another.

"I'D RATHER HAVE ROSES ON MY TABLE THAN DIAMONDS ON MY NECK."
— EMMA GOLDMAN

Dewy roses and powdery vanilla give a pomander a heavenly scent. Cover a foam ball with lunaria pods. Attach rosebuds by gluing together stems and poking them into the foam. Intersperse pink rose petals and tiny-leafed ivy sprays secured with florists pins. Mix 4 drops each of rose and vanilla oils; 2 drops geranium oil; and 1 drop jasmine oil, then apply to the foliage with an eye dropper. Use half, and save the rest for freshening.

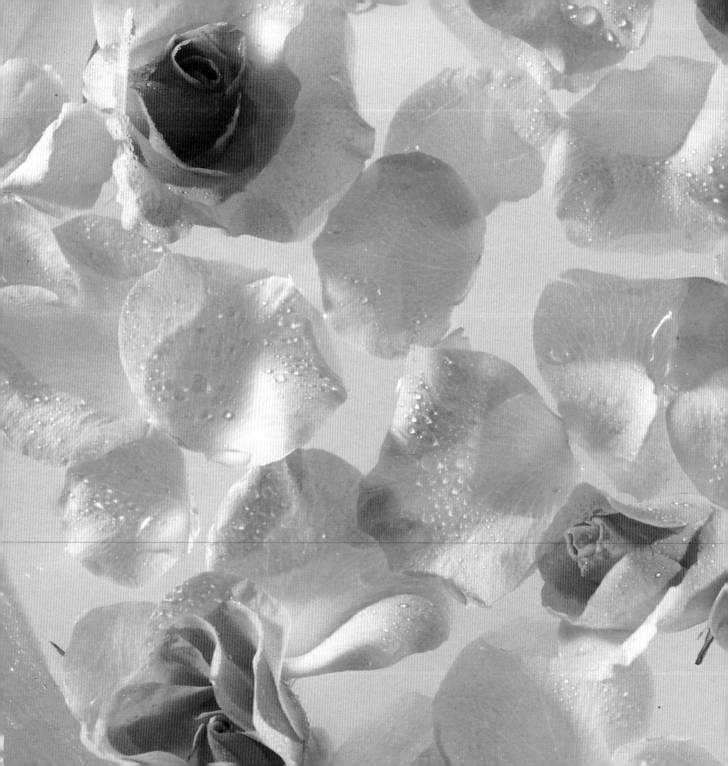

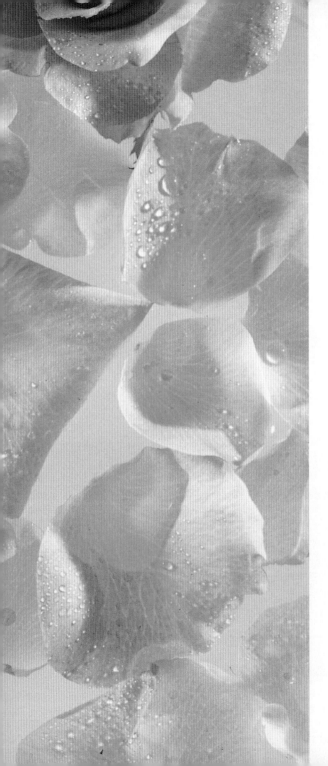

Herbal Rose Bath

1 cup chamomile

1 cup linden leaves

1 cup rose petals

1 cup catnip

The hydrating effect of roses, and the soothing effect of chamomile, make for an herbal bath that will soothe the nerves and pacify the mind.

Mix the herbs together in a large container. Pour 4 cups of boiling water over 1 cup of the mixture and let steep until cool. Strain and pour into the bath.

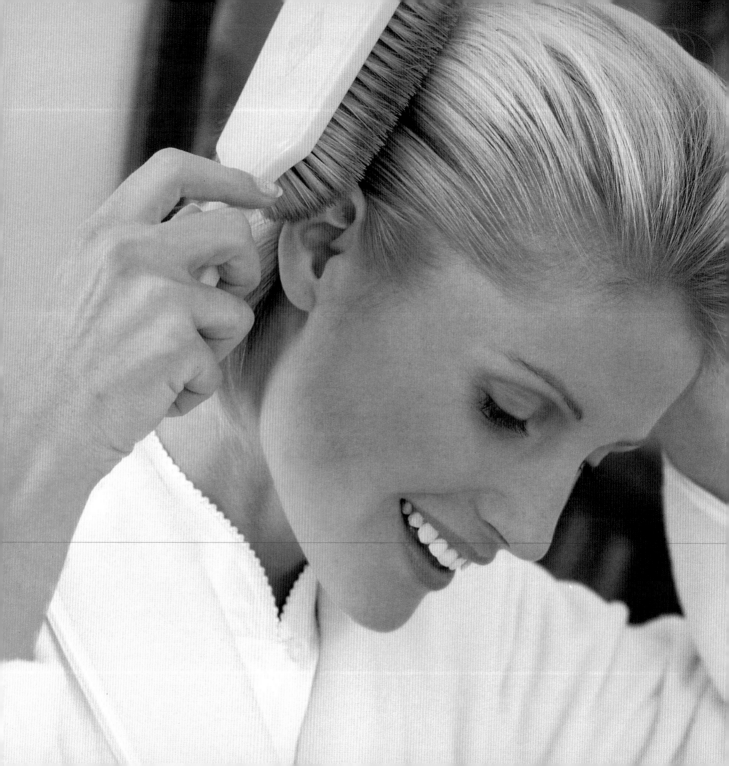

BEAUTY RITES
& RITUALS

When it comes to beauty, no part of it is as mysterious and confounding as styling hair. Perfect one morning, stubborn and unruly the next, your hair is fickle to its style, defiant to your will. A soft boar's-hair brush, an ivory comb—these are the beauty tools of time past. Oh, for the simplicity of it. Healthy, shiny hair comes from a good diet and proper care. A good style comes from a good cut, and using the right brush. Since there are hundreds to choose from, each built for a different hair type and end result, go to the source of your perfect hair day, your stylist. Ask your hairdresser to order the tools he or she uses on your locks so you can use them at home, or next time you're in the salon, get the style numbers and head for the nearest beauty supply store.

Today's arsenal of hair brushes includes styling tools to add volume and curl, and grooming brushes, which contain several kinds of natural bristles, to tame and add shine to the hair. Brushing hair should begin at the roots, not at the ends: Bend over and brush from the neckline. If you use a comb, select one that has wide teeth.

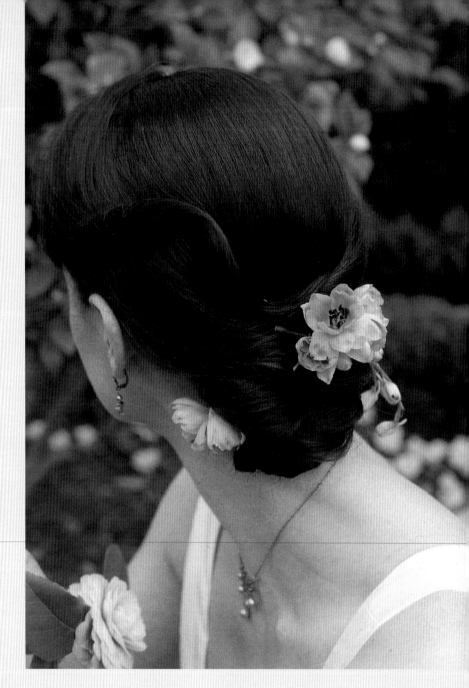

With a few fresh blossoms, artfully placed, your hair style can be transformed into an elegant and unforgettable one. Flowers should be the finishing touch, added just before you walk out the door to keep them from wilting. Beautifully made silk flowers, sprayed with your favorite perfume, can also be used to lend a touch of the season to your locks.

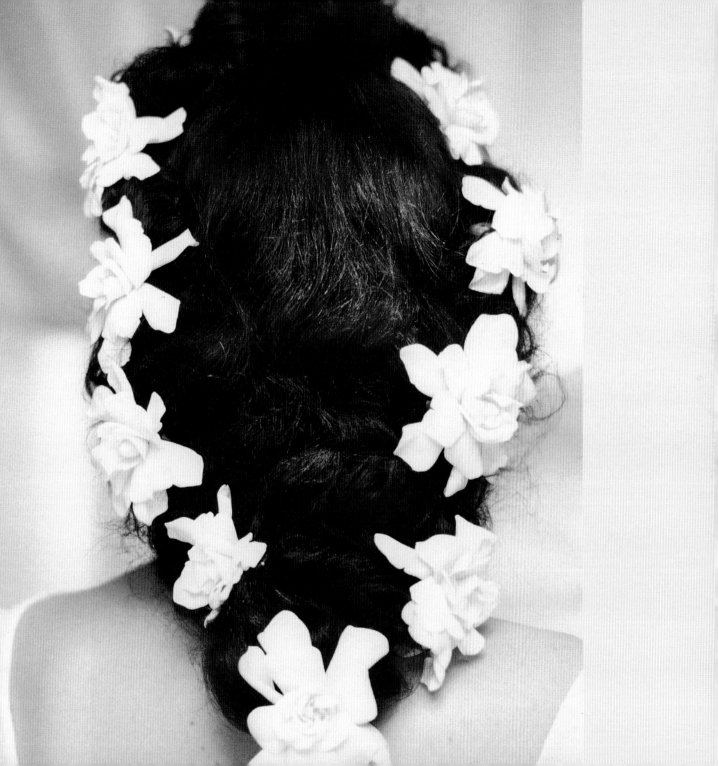

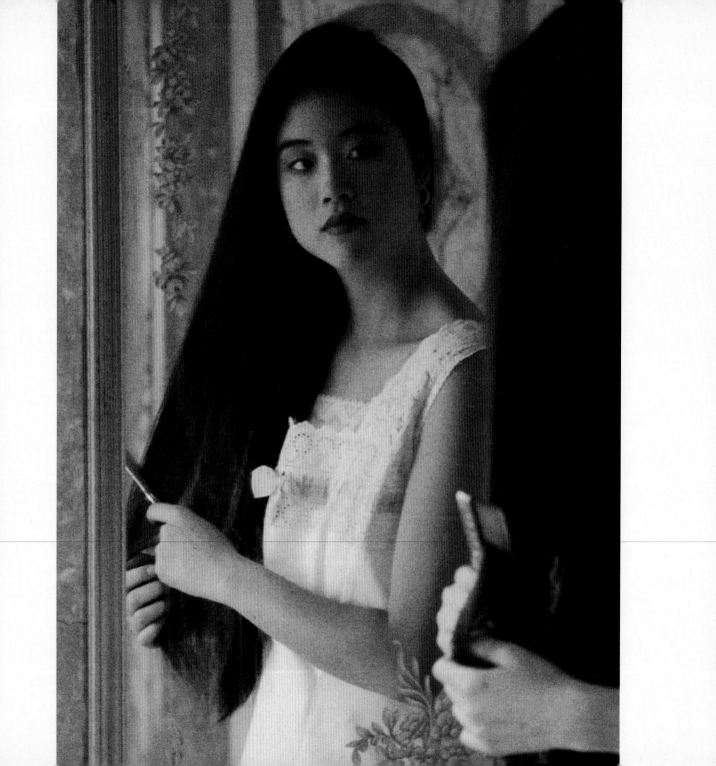

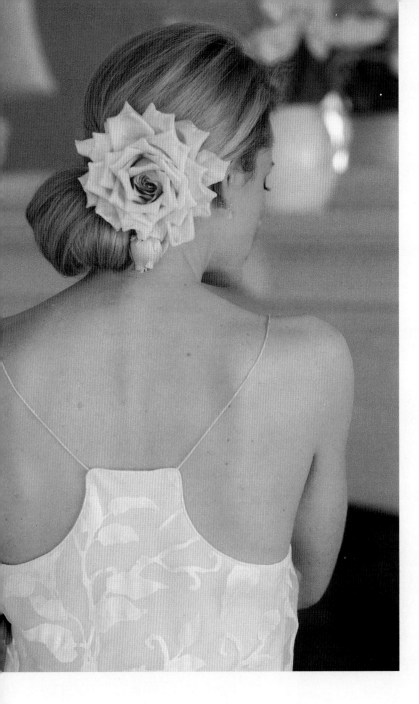

Summer
Rituals

Hair is rarely under your complete control, never less so than in summer. Golden sunbeams lighten your locks but can leave hair frizzy and dry. Hair craves the moisture in summer air, but humidity plays havoc with style. Changing the rules for your hair this season will help.

- Rinse instead of lather. When you rinse hair after playing in the ocean or pool, to prevent mineral buildup and access drying, just use water. Shampooing too frequently can strip hair of the natural oils that protect it.
- To remove mineral build-up, add a tablespoon of white vinegar to shampoo.
- Use conditioner to detangle hair so you're less apt to tug and break it. Conditioners also help lock moisture into hair.
- Pull back hair that's too unruly to tame, twist it and clip it.
- Get regular trims to maintain shape and remove frazzled ends.

ovely hands are, truly, poetry in motion. To grasp a loved one, touch the folds of crisp linen, massage oil into the skin, prepare a glorious meal—hands are our essential tools. Indeed, hands have a language all their own, known best by those who are closest to us. Caring for your hands is as important as taking care of your face.

The most essential part of hand and nail care is to moisturize them, which you should incorporate into a manicure. Keep manicures simple, and do them weekly to keep your fingers and cuticles well-groomed and healthy. First, soak fingers in warm water to soften nails before trimming. Gently file them with a fine-grained emery board, moving it only in one direction to avoid tearing nails.

Apply cuticle cream, then gently push back the dead skin on the nail towards cuticles. (Never cut cuticles as this risks infection and hangnails.) As a final touch, massage a moisturizer in and around nails. Keep a cuticle treatment on hand and apply frequently (especially after doing the dishes).

DAILY RITUAL

Indian dancers use this exercise to strengthen fingers and make hands more expressive: Holding your hand upright, bend your thumb into your palm and slowly lower your fingers over the thumb one at a time, then raise your fingers, starting with the pinkie, one at a time. Shake out your hand and repeat several times.

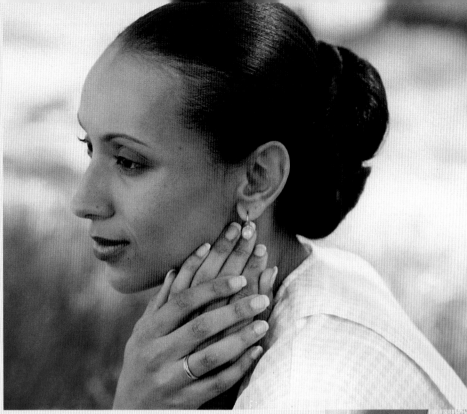

Chipped, brittle, peeling
nails can be temporarily for-
tified by polish-like treatments until they grow out,
but to avoid such a condition
in the first place, you should
apply hand cream or another
moisturizer both in the
morning and at night. For
a feel-good and beneficial
nail massage, soak fingers
in warmed olive oil, then
massage the oil into the
nail area.

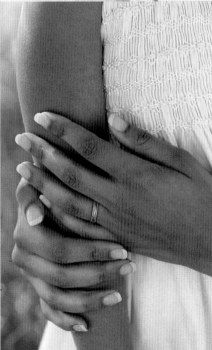

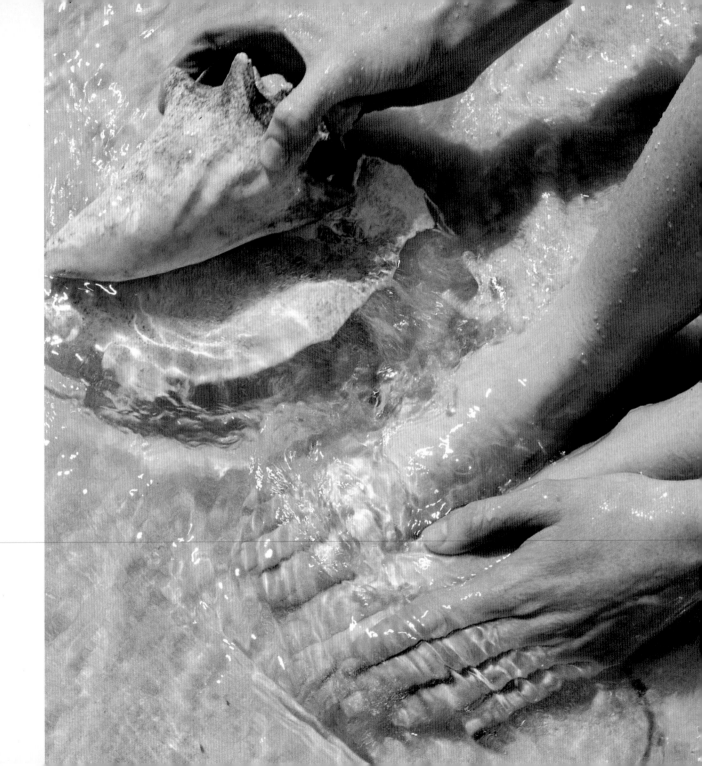

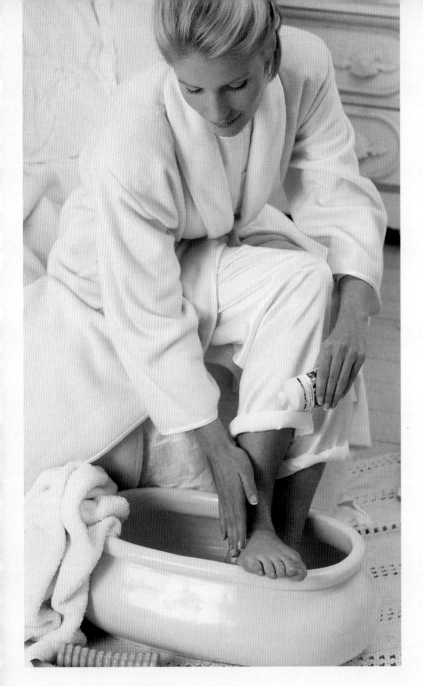

Feet are considered the body's most responsive area for accessing energy zones. Reflexologists believe the entire body is mapped on the feet, starting with the toes to reflect the head. A foot massage is said to stimulate 7,000 nerves.

- The perfect pedicure should begin with a foot soak in warm water.

- Add Epsom salts to relieve inflammation, or essential oils for aromatherapeutic benefits.

- Remove rough skin with a pumice stone or a cream that contains exfoliating granules.

- Moisturize with a thick pomade, paying special attention to heels and toenails.

- Apply cuticle cream and gently push back cuticles with a towel or manicure stick.

- Trim toenails straight across; avoid filing the corners, which can cause ingrown toenails. Smooth with an emery board.

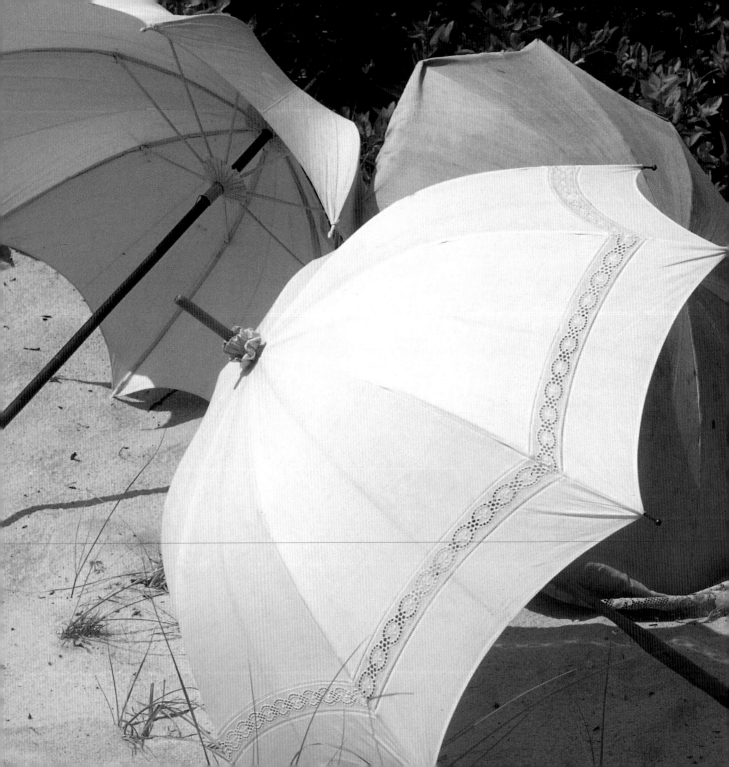

To weave sun and shade: this is the challenge of summer months. The sun's light can burn and prematurely age your skin. To prevent this, consider wearing a hat with a wide brim; it is the best way to shield your delicate face, neck, ears, and eyes. (Drape a simple straw hat with lace fichu or a swath of netting to add romance to your walk under midday rays.) Bring an umbrella outdoors so that you will not be exposed to the sun all day long.

Religiously follow these guidelines to protect against the sun's ravages:

- Wear sunglasses that block ultraviolet rays, both UVA and UVB.
- Choose tightly woven, loose-fitting clothing.
- Always wear a sunscreen with the Sun Protection Factor (SPF) 15 or higher. If you're playing, working, or exercising, reapply it every two hours.
- Limit your exposure to the sun between 10AM and 2PM, when rays are strongest.
- Protect the children and teenagers in your life. Researchers know that although the sun's damaging effects do not show up until later in life, the majority of most people's sun exposure occurs before age twenty.

"I HAVE NOT YET GROWN WEARY OF LOOKING AT THE WATER, DOING NOTHING, THINKING IDLY IN A HAPHAZARD SORT OF WAY."
—DORIS GRUMBACH

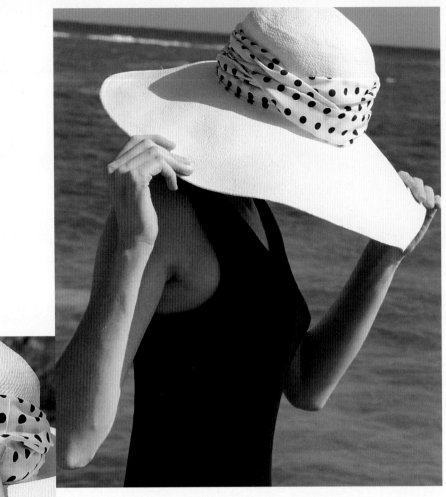

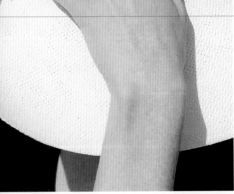

The best sun block is shade—and a hat offers unparalleled protection. Because they are available in such a variety of styles, hats are easy to incorporate into your summer wardrobe. What we consider the signs of aging—wrinkles, leathery skin texture, blotches—come not from getting older, but from sun exposure. Skin that is shielded from the sun's damaging rays—regard your inner arm—stays soft and supple, even as the years pass.

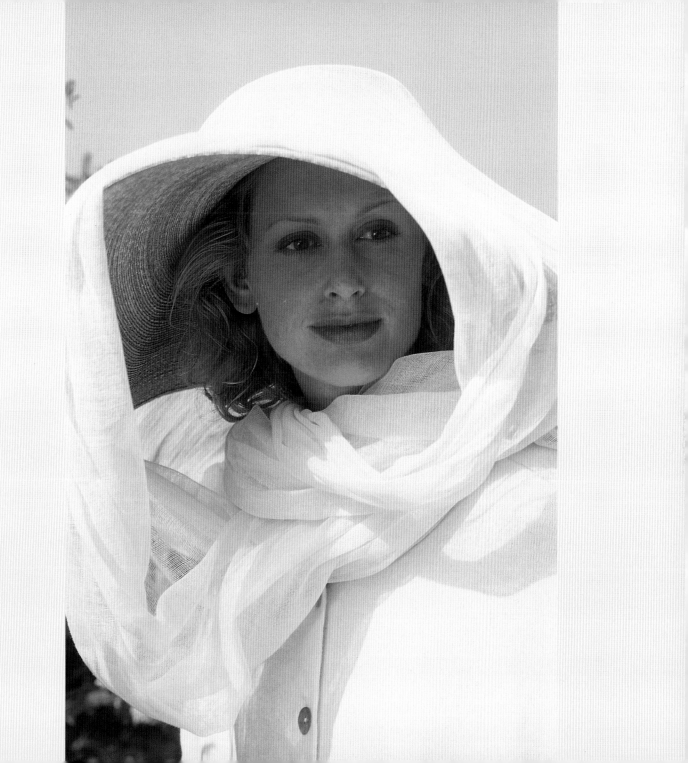

Pleasure of *Scent*

Calendula
Massage Oil

1/3 cup calendula

2 cups almond oil

Yellow-flowered calendula—marigold—is a hardy annual that thrives in the sun. It is a natural healer and has many therapeutic uses, especially in summertime: it is a good antidote to bruises and bug bites.

Place the calendula in the almond oil and steep in a glass jar, covered, for two weeks in the sun. Use the mixture at full strength.

An astringent can also be made with calendula: Place the herb in a bottle of cider vinegar and let steep, covered, for two weeks. Dilute the astringent with an equal amount of water before using.

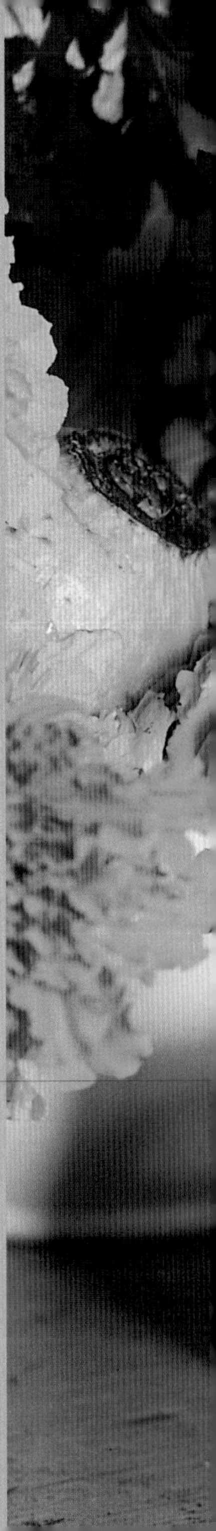

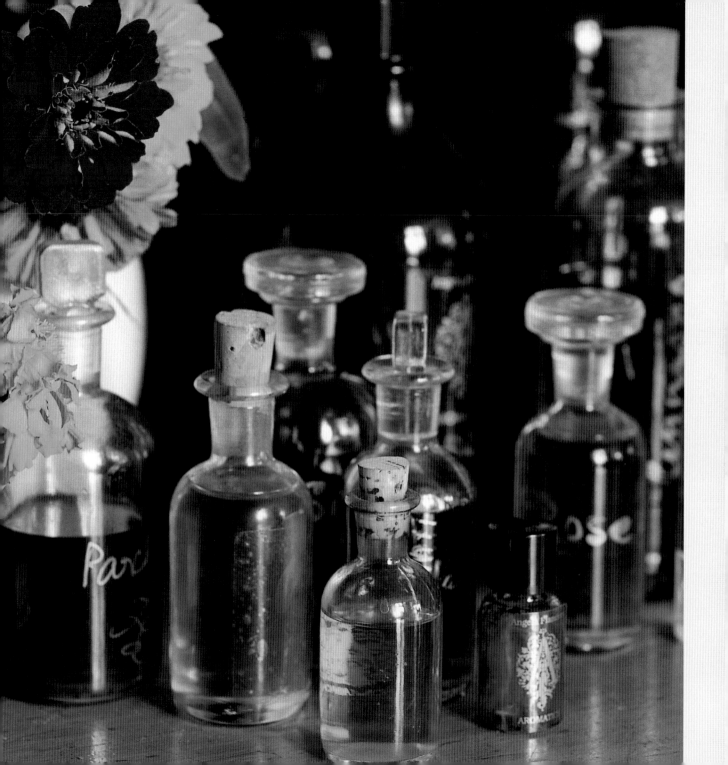

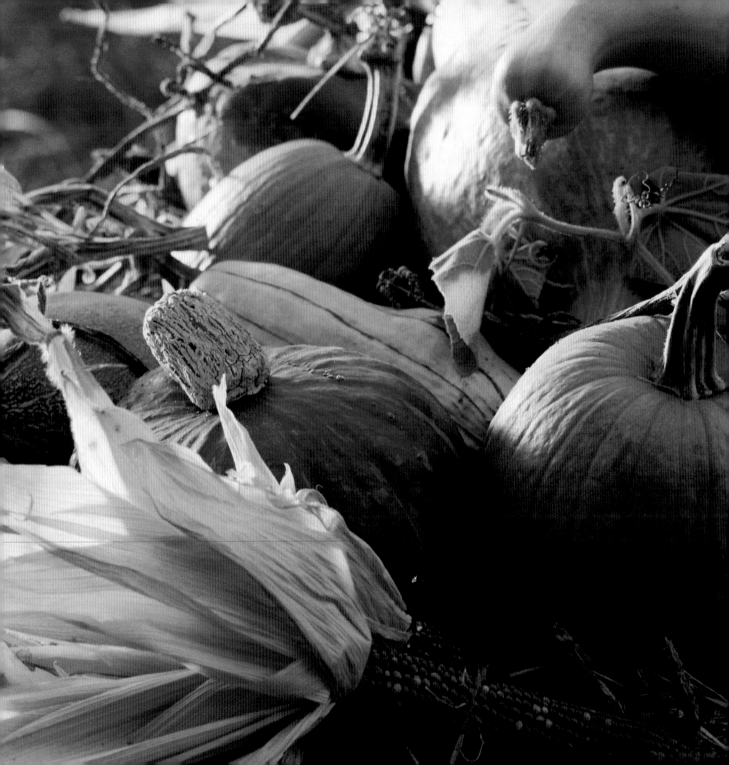

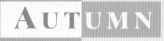

Autumn

Natural colors

Natural colors

Just as each life follows its own course, autumn follows summer. There is something about shorter days and crisper nights, brilliant yellow gingko leaves against the sky, fragrant apples in a crate, a field of resting pumpkins, that can bring your heart to your throat. Melancholy for some who hate to bid summer farewell, busy for many as schools open and holidays loom, autumn is nevertheless an exciting time of change. The possibilities can seem endless. Nature's offerings—of jewel-toned flowers, finally ripe fruits, scarlet, orange, and golden foliage—provide proof that visible change inevitably follows life's quiet, invisible work, and that it is exhilarating. Fall offers a cornucopia of riches that beautify: nuts used in oils to smooth the skin; rose hips and witch hazel included in toners and skin fresheners; scents of cedar and figs found in fragrances. Nature's autumn hues, earthy and bright, from bark to cranberry, inspire the new shades at the cosmetic counters. Be open to change, let the outside in, make this season, too often called off-season, your own. Take a brisk walk on the beach, dressed warmly; jog, run, go exuberantly into fall.

EXUBERANCE IS BEAUTY.
—WILLIAM BLAKE

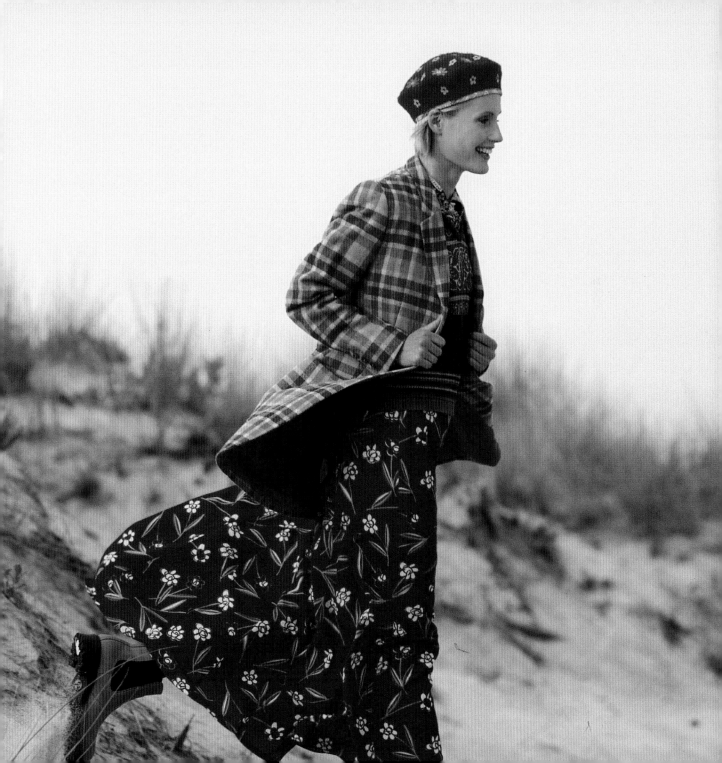

A Place for Beauty

The era of the large, lavish Victorian bathroom—which was outfitted with furniture and accessories like any other room in the house—came to an end with the introduction of the five-foot long tub, around which bathrooms began to be sized. As it became possible and affordable to install bathrooms in every home, bathroom fittings became simpler and more functional. But the detail and elegance of those sumptuous Victorian bathrooms need not be lost. In the fall, when life moves back indoors, revisit the bathroom and endow it with something beautiful—a new mirror, a dressing table, a set of drawers.

Dressing tables harbor the secrets and longings of our femininity, whether it's an elaborate antique *poudresse* with tiny drawers, or a simple table with a marble top.

"IT WAS A WARM SEPTEMBER MORNING, AGLOW WITH MELLOW SUNLIGHT . . . WITH LEAVES FLUTTERING IN THE WIND."
—W. PHILIP KELLER

The place we choose to pursue beauty need not be particularly fancy or elaborate—a little nook will do, so long as the light is true and essentials are kept well-organized and close at hand.

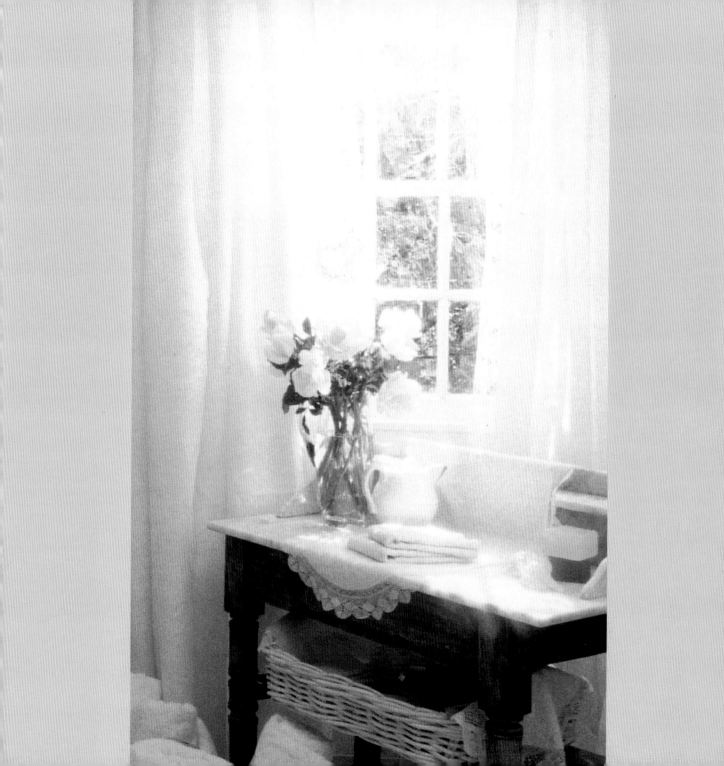

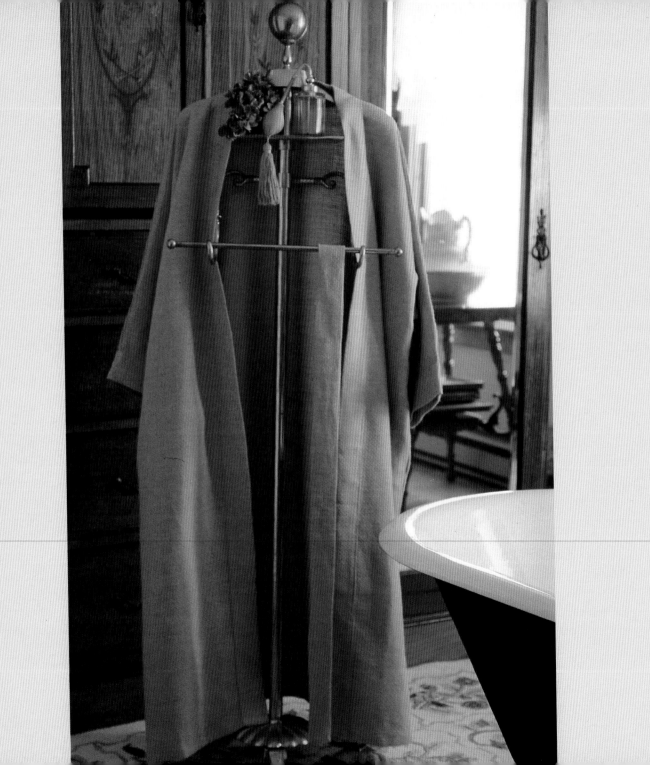

They've been a part of our daily beauty routine for three centuries, and women have long struggled to keep them clear. In fall, the season of experiencing a new cosmetic palette, dressing table surfaces can become crowded, camouflaging what you need. Hints on staying clutter-free: Keep like things together; use baskets to separate makeup brushes from eyeshadows, eyelash curlers from lotions. Throw out anything you haven't touched in six months or that you've had for over two years.

VINTAGE LINENS

Vintage linens and lace create a distinctly romantic mood in a bathroom, but keeping them clean can be a challenge. Before washing any antique cloth, especially one with colored embroidery, check with a restoration expert to see if it should be laundered at all. If your treasure will withstand a water wash, follow these steps:

- Before washing, remove metal fasteners that might discolor the fabric.
- Place the fabric in cool or lukewarm water combined with a cleaning solution made for vintage fabrics. Let the fabric soak; do not wring or rub it.
- As the water becomes dirty, change it, adding fresh cleaner as necessary.
- Soaps and cleansers can leave residue that can weaken fabric, so your final rinse should happen in several stages. After each rinse of fresh water, lift the fabric out of the water holding its underside, not the edges.
- Blot the fabric with towels and place it flat on a dry towel or sheet to dry.
- Gently press it with a fresh towel to blot moisture and properly shape it.
- Press, using a low heat setting on the iron and a pressing cloth. Lace may not need pressing; embroidered pieces should be placed face down on a towel.

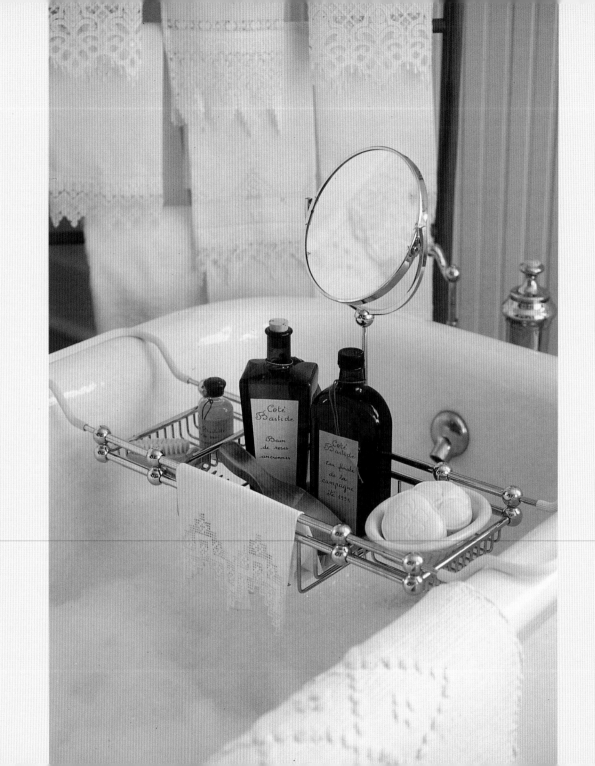

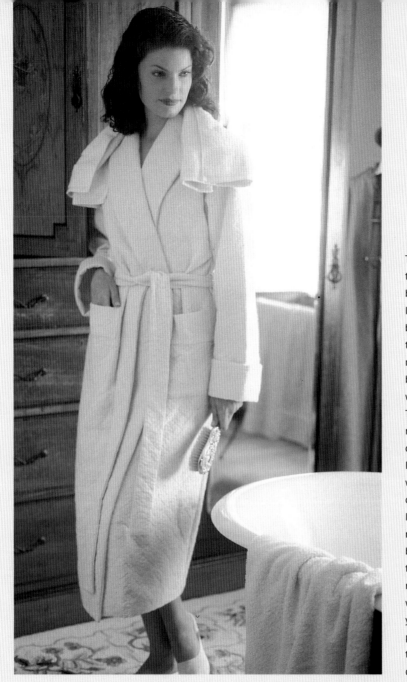

The bathroom can be transformed into a place of beauty with elements both large and small. A simple bath tray (opposite) holds the necessities of bathing: a mirror for facial masques, bottles of fragrant bath waters, hand-milled soap. The chrome edges of the room are softened by delicate lace towels. Outfit a large bathroom with a wooden dresser (left), which can hold extra towels and linens, taken from another room in the house. In all bathrooms, the important thing is to create an unhurried, comfortable place where you can contemplate your day, nurture and pamper yourself, and complete the finishing touches of the dressing ritual.

The act of self-regard—of looking at one's own reflection—has been a part of human behavior since Narcissus first leaned over that pool of water. In ancient times, people peered into mirrors made of polished metals; then, in the 1600s, mirrors of silvered glass appeared. Because glass mirrors were small and quite expensive, heavy, elaborate frames were built around them to enhance their impact.

The possibilities for mirrors in the bathroom might include a handheld mirror that is easily transportable and a "cheval glass" mirror, usually of full-figure length and set between vertical posts (a smaller version is made to be placed upon a dressing table). Modern makeup and shaving mirrors make daily routines easier and more enhancing, especially with proper lighting. Antique mirrors add a matchless sense of history and charm to a bathroom, but if it's the clearest reflection in the world you want, install a new glass in the old frame. Skin colors will be truest in mirrors labeled "ultra-clear," which contain less iron than other mirrors, reducing a greenish tint. In damp areas, mirrors made the traditional way, with chemicals called silvering, can corrode. Look for mirrors made with the pyrolytic process to hang in bathrooms.

"I HAVE SOMETIMES THOUGHT THAT A WOMAN'S NATURE IS LIKE A GREAT HOUSE, FULL OF ROOMS. —EDITH WHARTON

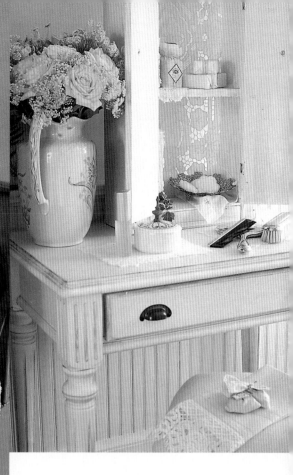

A lady going abroad was sure to travel with a complete vanity case. Elegant turn-of-the-century versions like this one (left), complete with its original enameled hand mirrors, are still prized by travelers, and make a charming touch in a guest room. A clutter-free vanity table (above) makes preparing for the day a pleasure.

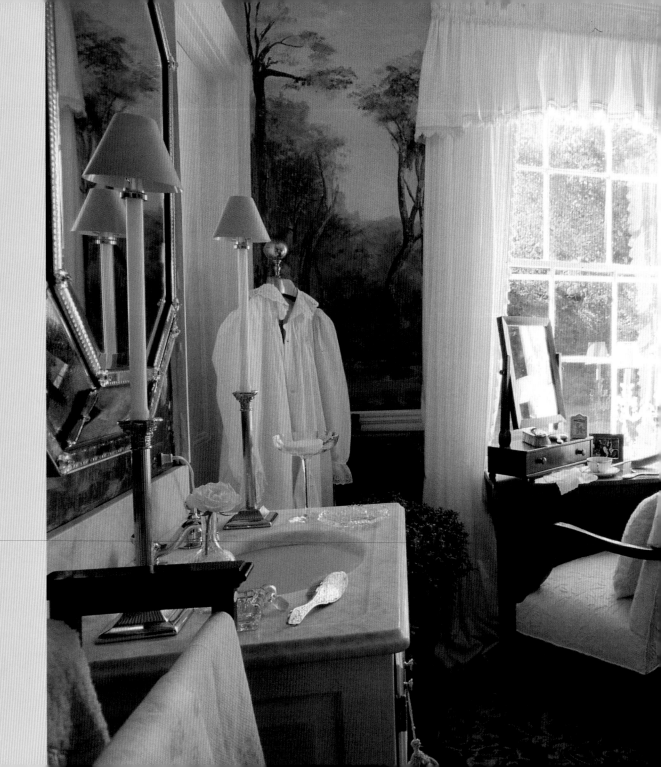

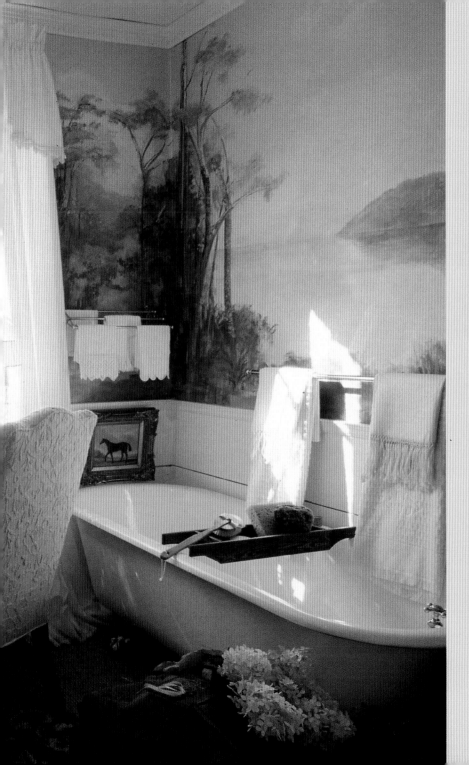

A meditative moment can be had in a bathroom designed for everyday necessities as well as flights of fancy. Here, in a tribute to the well-equipped Victorian bathroom, a New England lolling chair, 18th-century dressing table, and mural that invites daydreams all contribute to a grand sense of privacy and retreat.

Moments of Meditation

The hallmark of autumn is change, from the leaves in your garden to the feast on your table; from a "back-to-school" wardrobe to an updated haircut or shade of lipstick. But as long as the stresses and worries of daily life are exhausting you, inner change is impossible. Stress management experts say dealing with tension has three dimensions: Changing stressful conditions, which could be anything from reorganizing your pantry to finding a new job; changing negative thought patterns, which means turning off your inner-critic and replacing belittling inner monologues with non-judgmental messages, and finally, incorporating relaxation techniques into your daily life.

Once mastered, consistent acts of relaxation and meditation have physical as well as psychological benefits: Health-care professionals advocate meditation to

While traditional meditation calls for sitting still in silence, activities like gardening, manicuring your nails, playing an instrument, or simply walking can also be considered meditative, as long as your mind is quiet.

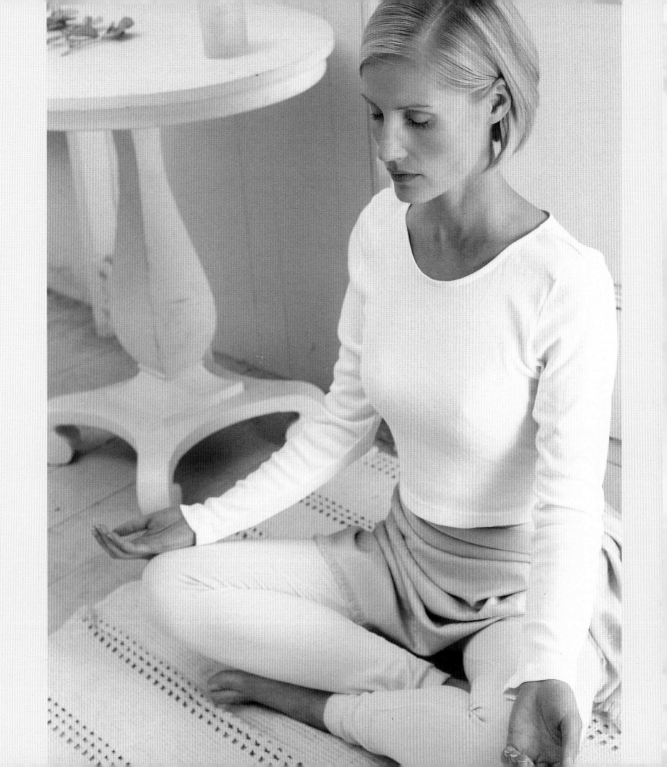

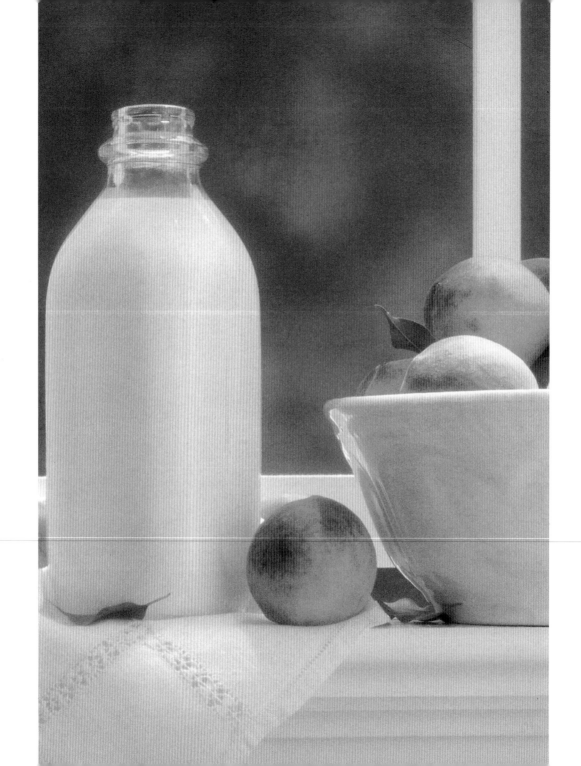

lower blood-pressure and to help with depression, chronic infections, pain, and high cholesterol.

Just ten minutes of meditation a day can be enough to relax you. There are several ways to meditate. If you have never tried it before, a good way to start is to sit comfortably, close your eyes, and count four slow, even breaths over and over until several minutes have passed. Let images or thoughts arise as they will, but view them with detachment, letting them drift in and out of your consciousness like clouds. Keep counting, focusing on the breath. At first, sitting this way for three minutes may feel like eons. But with practice, your breathing and ability to empty your mind will become easier. Once you have mastered the basics, you may want to investigate deeper levels of meditation, include visualization techniques, or explore an activity that incorporates meditation, such as yoga.

AS AUTUMN MARCHES
TOWARDS WINTER
MEDITATE IN A MILK BATH
AND HEAL DRY SKIN

Few at-home remedies are as perfect as milk, which contains proteins, vitamins, and minerals that are absorbed by the skin. A milk bath moisturizes and heals dry, itchy skin at the same time it offers you an escape from your hectic fall schedule. After showering, add 2 cups of powdered milk and 2 cups of fresh whole milk to a warm bath, along with 6 to 10 drops of your favorite essential oil. Soak for 20 minutes, towel dry, and apply moisturizer.

GIFT OF NATURE

"SMELL IS A POTENT WIZARD THAT TRANSPORTS US, ACROSS THOUSANDS OF MILES AND ALL THE YEARS WE HAVE LIVED."
—HELEN KELLER

Our noses have the ability to recognize about 10,000 different smells, and while every person responds differently to them, there seem to be a few universals. In fall, some of the heady pleasures of the season come from cavorting through leaves or taking a woodland walk and breathing in deeply the fragrances that feed the soul—the acrid scent of burning leaves, the sweet smells of home-made applesauce, roasted turkey, pumpkin pie. On your walks, pick up pinecones for a potpourri; select botanicals for fall fragrances from a health-food store. Woody scents like cinnamon (believed to be an aphrodisiac), sandalwood (its rich and sweet scent is exquisite in blends), and cloves (spicy and refreshing) are good ones to consider this season.

The Victorians were among the first to embellish pewter, adding decorative touches to the rustic vessels that were the mainstays of Welsh cupboards. The cinnamon, spicy aroma of mulled cider in a pewter tankard expresses November's warm welcome to family and friends.

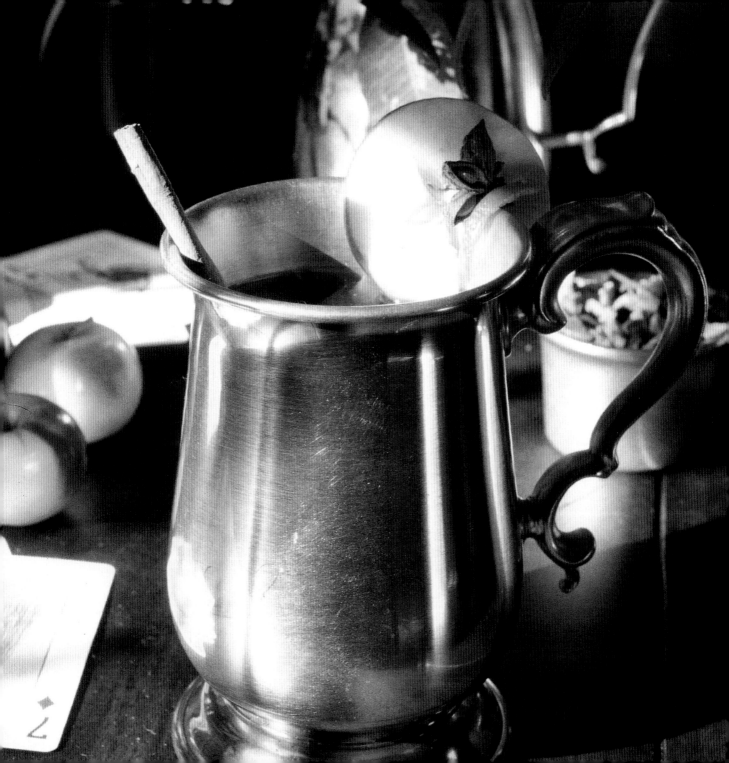

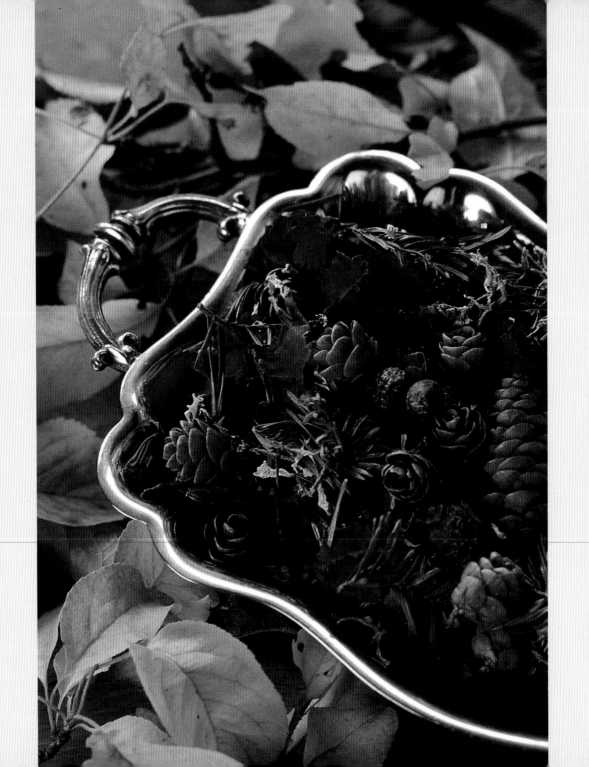

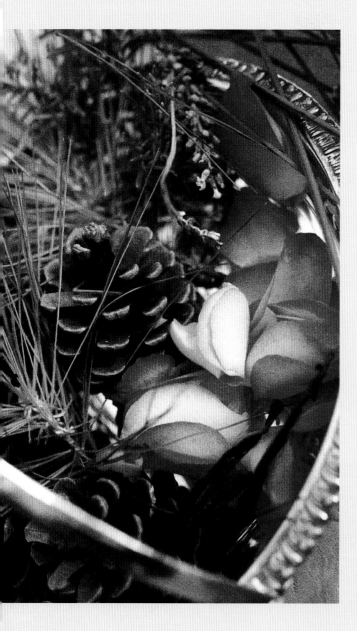

AUTUMN LEAVES POTPOURRI

2 cups mixed rose hips, rose petals, and rose leaves

1 cup sweet woodruff

1/2 cup lavender

1/4 cup each: juniper berries, sandalwood, rosemary, oak-moss, tansy or myrtle leaves

1 tsp. cloves

1 cup mixed pine needles and pinecones

1/2 vanilla bean

1 handful birch or scented geranium leaves

8 drops bayberry oil

10 drops vanilla oil

10 drops rose oil

3 drops blue-spruce oil

Dried autumn leaves for color

Mix all the leaves and flowers first, then add the drops of oil. Red and orange maple, or brown oak and yellow sassafras leaves add wonderful color to the blend.

BEAUTY RITES & RITUALS

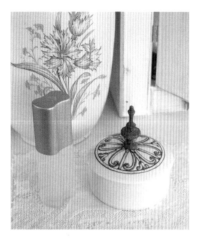

In fall, senses are piqued, and it is a good time to re-evaluate your beauty choices. Cosmetics counters offer a new season's bounty—different shades of makeup and unique fragrances, each with its own allure. Be open to revisions. Too easily, makeup artists say, we tend to stay with makeup hues we've always worn, disregarding how our faces have changed over time. So, take a moment to reflect on your reflection. Find the features you want to emphasize (taking care not to choose them all). And seek out the makeup shades, hair cut, or color that best fit the face in the mirror, not the face in your mind.

The most important aspects of your beauty routine are the thoughts and feelings you have about yourself. For many women passing seasons don't necessarily mean

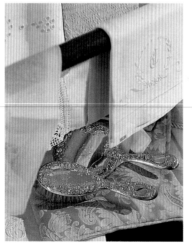

Condition your hands with a hand soak: apply moisturizer, then immerse them in very hot water. As desired, add 2 tablespoons of sea salt and 6 to 8 drops of essential oils: peppermint and rosemary to refresh and stimulate; tea tree and lavender to relax and heal; sandalwood and chamomile to soothe. After the soak, reapply moisturizer.

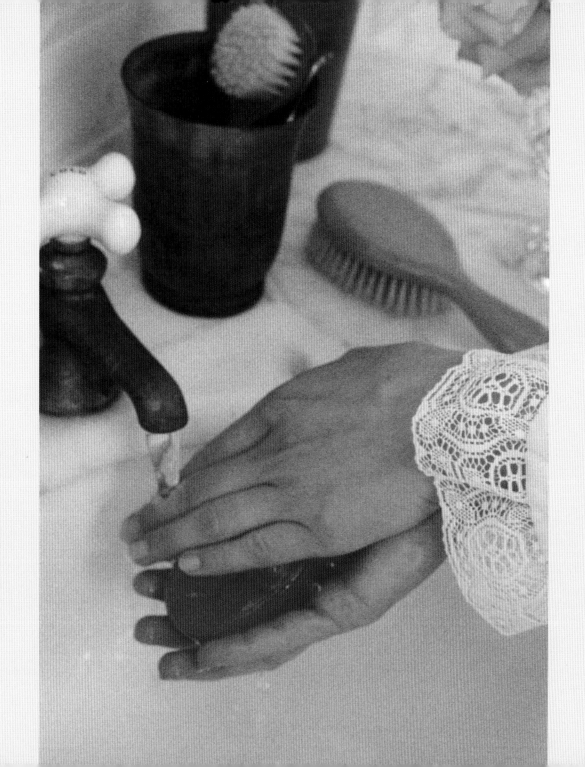

wiser self-images. Body-image experts note that women often fall into the trap of repeating self-criticisms, even those from childhood. To battle that, therapists advocate exercises to help lose the negative monologue. One such classic: jot down unpleasant comments you make about your appearance, without judging them. Afterwards, spend five minutes looking in the mirror, making a mental note of the features you're happy with. You'll probably find the notes you scribble down don't have anything to do with what you see in the mirror.

As for fall makeup, leave sheer, bronzed (with makeup or self-tanner) faces behind, and achieve a natural look with foundation, powder, and blush. Before you apply any powder or blush, you'll need to find the perfect foundation. The most natural shades have brown, beige, or yellow undertones and will disappear into your skin if you've matched it correctly. (Orange- and pink-based foundations are more apt to give you a mask-like look.) Foundations are formulated to work not only with skin tone but also with skin type. Every type can use liquid makeup; dry skin works well with creme-based foundations. Tinted moisturizer offers minimum coverage, but offers a healthy glow without a makeup feel.

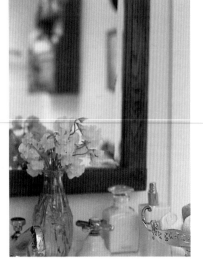

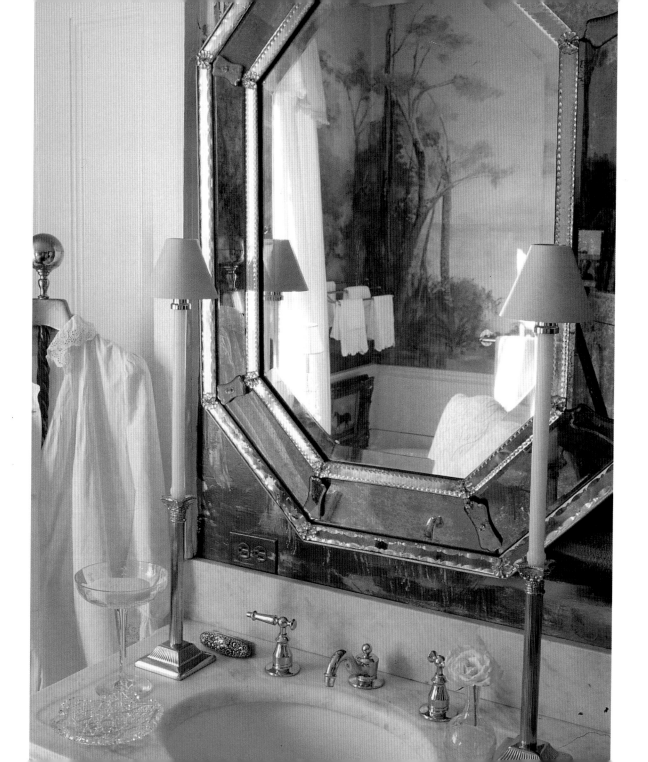

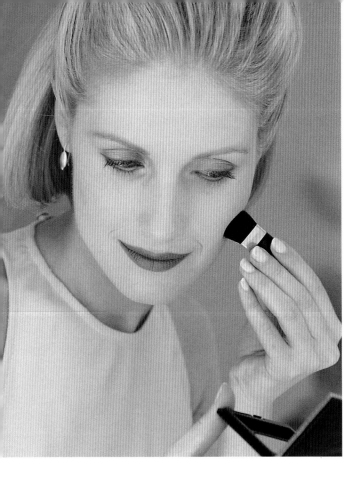

"THE MOST BEAUTIFUL
MAKEUP OF A WOMAN
IS PASSION.
BUT COSMETICS ARE
EASIER TO BUY."
—YVES ST. LAURENT

DAILY RITUAL

Applying blush is not an art, but it is sometimes approached as one. It can be tricky to find the apples in your cheeks, but trying too hard—creating cheekbones with blush—almost always looks fake. Generally, creme blushes work best on dry skin; powders on oilier skins. Use a blush brush to lightly apply color over the cheekbones and blend in a circular motion.

Pressed powder is good for touch-ups; all other times, use loose powder. Applied lightly with a brush, powder provides a smooth, "finished" look. It helps even skin tone, cuts down shine, and, when used under eye shadow and lipstick, will help keep makeup on.

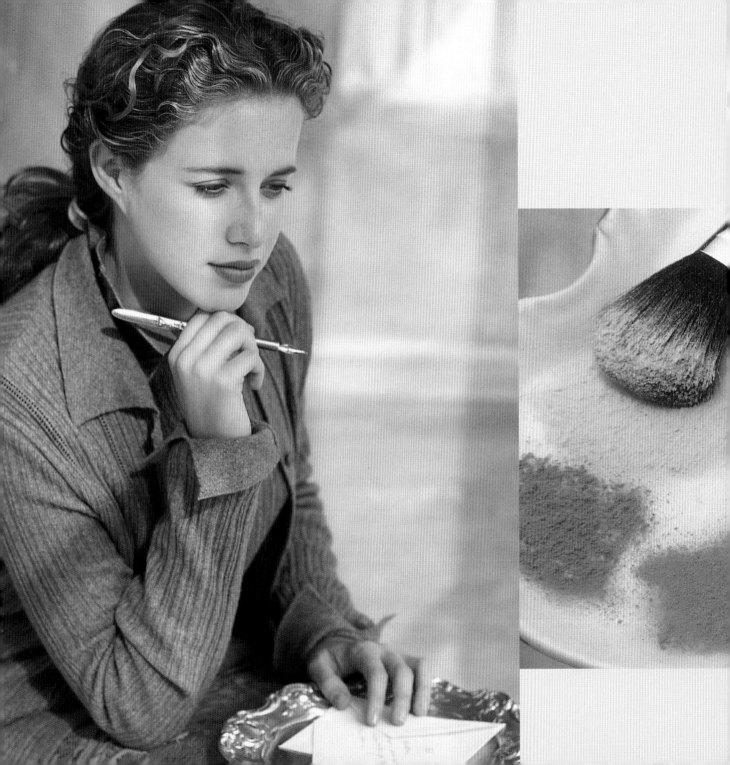

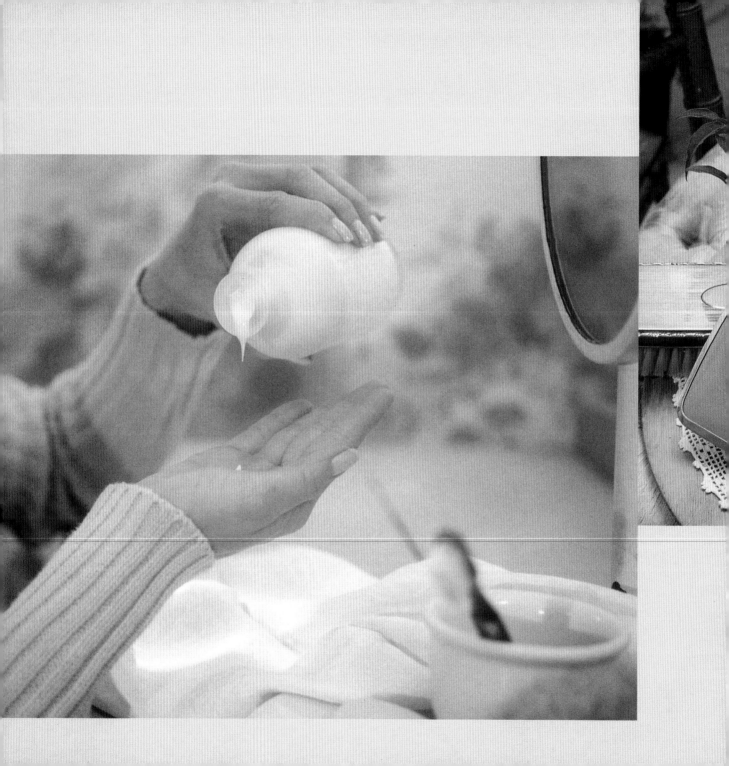

The basics of caring for one-self can include a simple hand lotion (opposite), a mirror (above), and fine soaps (right). Whether or not your tastes include collecting antique items of vanity such as Staffordshire bowls decorated with cherubs, consider these words from the poet Hui-Hai, "Your treasure house is within, it contains all you'll ever need."

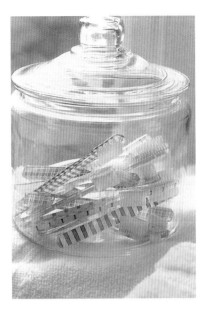

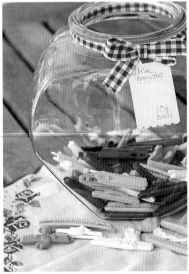

We may take it for granted that the creams and makeup we put on our face are safe, and we should. (The practice of using white lead in makeup to whiten faces ended in the nineteenth century.) But even though there is nothing in makeup today that will harm you, if a product isn't made with the correct preservatives or is not stored properly, bacteria can build up and may increase your likelihood of getting an infection. To maintain the quality of your cosmetics, follow these precautions:

- Store products out of sunlight.
- Keep containers tightly sealed when not in use.
- Never share makeup—and don't use testers at the counter; insist on a fresh applicator.
- Don't use eye makeup if you have an eye infection, and toss all products you were using when you first discovered the infection.
- Never add water or liquid to a product to bring it back to its original consistency.
- Throw away cosmetics if the color changes or an odor develops.

Glass jars (left) and an old apothecary cabinet (opposite) gain new life as receptacles for beauty. Clearly labeled and organized beauty products can be as much a design element in a bathroom as a necessity.

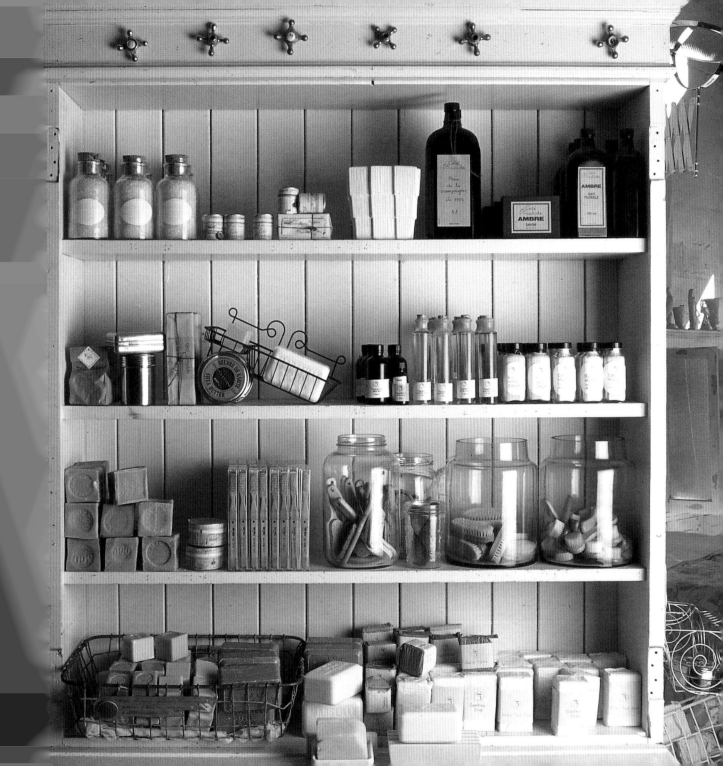

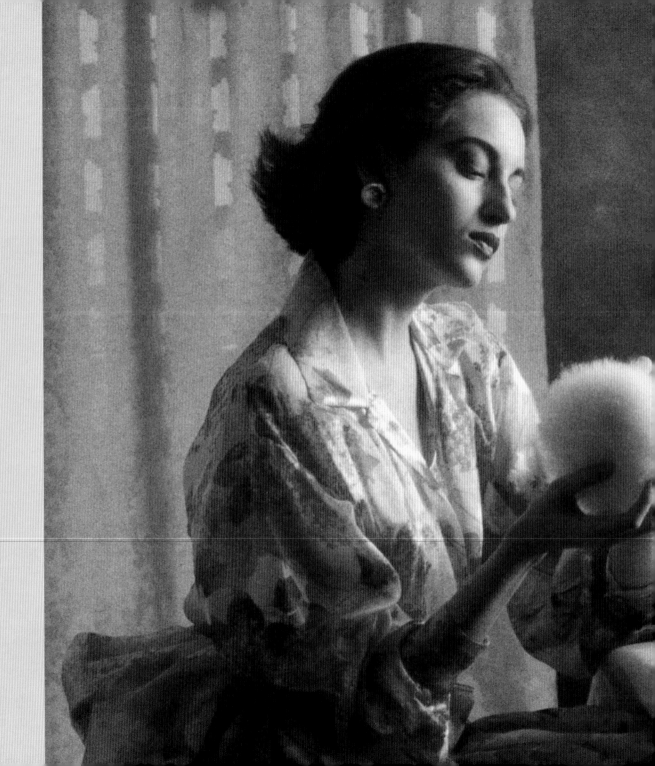

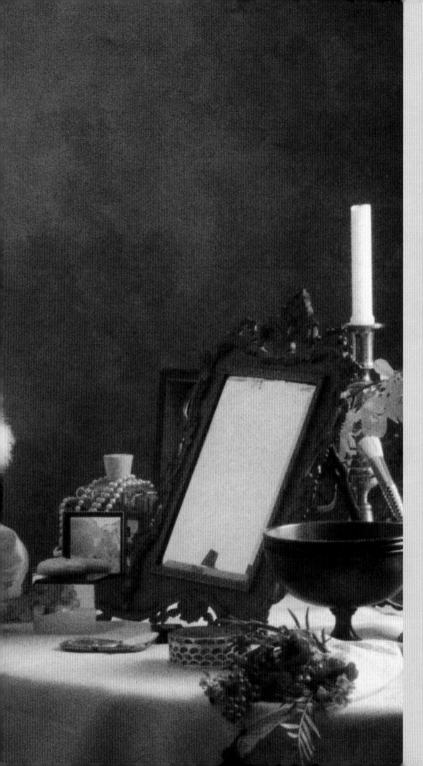

Autumn Rituals

The season to be out in the evening—at soirees, balls, and other occasions—beckons. This is a time to wear a slightly more glamorous look and to remember ways to keep makeup staying put.

- Play up eyes, cheeks or lips, not all features or your face will look over-done. Simplicity is the key.
- Deepen your eye makeup with smoky shadows and pencils.
- Wear stronger red or burgundy lip color.
- Use lip gloss.
- Use transparent powder to give your face a finished look.
- Keep eye shadow from creasing or caking by using loose powder on your eyelids after applying eye makeup.
- To help keep lipstick in place, apply lip liner first, then top with lipstick.

Pleasure of Scent

Invigorating Bath Soak

¹/4 cup lemon verbena

¹/4 cup thyme

¹/4 cup chamomile

¹/4 cup mint

rind of 1 lemon

When the busy rush of the fall season drains your energy, try this exhilarating bath soak. It contains lemon, which stimulates and uplifts, and mint, which energizes the spirit. The chamomile will help to calm any frayed nerves.

Tie the herbs in a small muslin bag or in a handkerchief, and hang them from the bath spigot while filling the tub. Let the bag soak in the water while you are bathing, then finish by rubbing the bag all over your body before you towel dry.

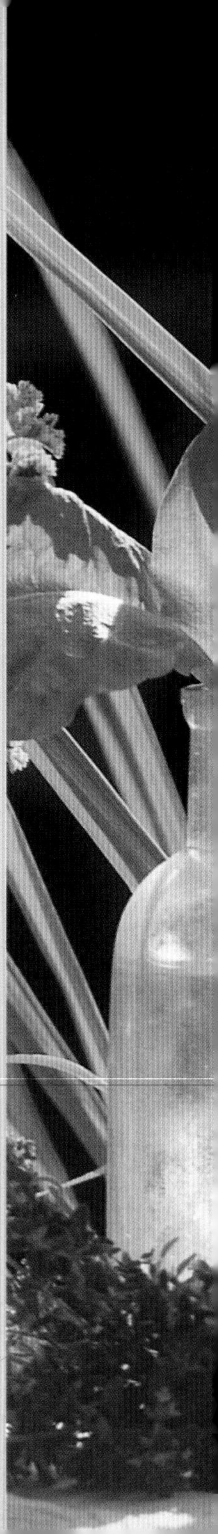

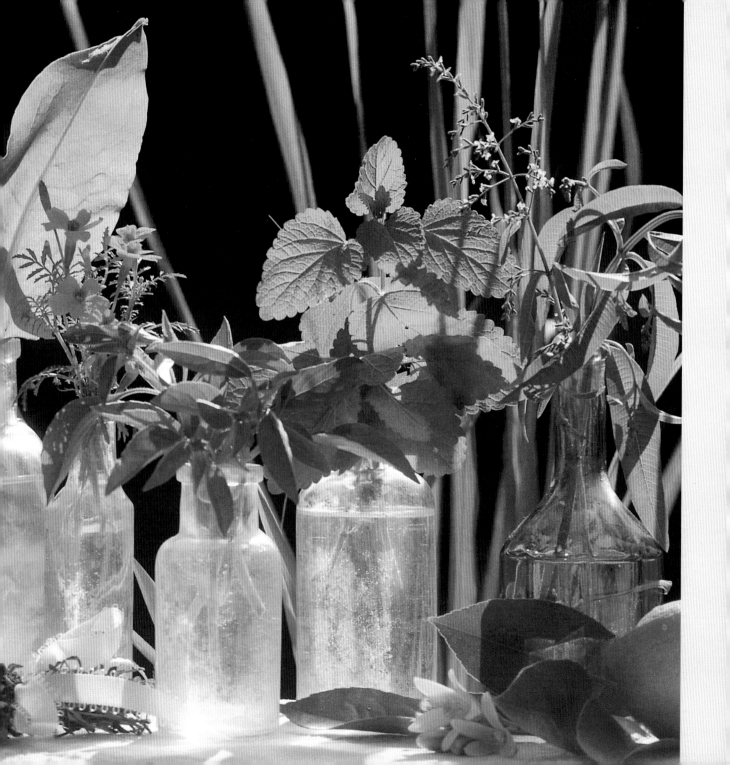

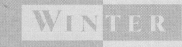

Dusting of powder

Dusting of powder

Winter is energizing in its duality. It is a quiet season of early twilight, a time of indoor reflection and peace; at the same time it means preparing for the busy splendors of Hanukkah, Christmas, Kwanzaa, and the New Year celebration. The memories formed in winter—and the scents that accompany them—stay with you a lifetime: wood fires, fragrant ovens, soaked mittens, hyacinths on the windowsill. As temperatures drop and skies are brittle blue, winter also commands you to bundle up and step outside. It is the time to experience, as Anne Morrow Lindbergh wrote, many climates of feeling in one day. As you shop for your loved ones, prepare traditional meals, make gifts, send cards—all the while reflecting on the past year and preparing for a new one—tend to your own inner self. In this busy season, your beauty regimens can too often become rote or put on hold. Take the time to be present in your daily rituals. The cleansing of your face, each shower or bath, presents an opportunity to let your mind mine its own inner workings.

ALL FREEZES AGAIN—
AMONG THE PINES,
WINDS WHISPERING
A PRAYER.

— RIEI, 18TH-CENTURY
JAPANESE POET

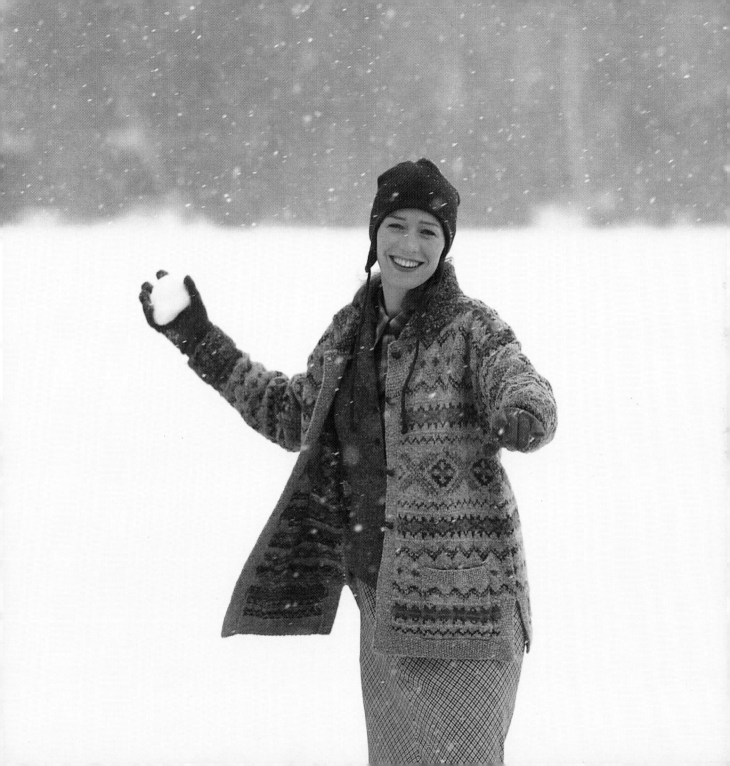

To Greet a Guest

In winter, our homes fill with guests—longtime friends, close family, children and their roommates back from college. It has always been a time to indulge those we love, to shower them with little treats. A bathroom reserved for visitors may be considered a luxury, but it is an especially inviting retreat for winter travelers. And with a few thoughtful gestures even a small powder room can be transformed into a soothing oasis, a place for visitors to collect their thoughts.

You can create a welcoming mood in a bathroom by adding your own personal touches. Group candles for an atmosphere of serenity and light; display colorful bath beads and oils, or place bath salts in a shell—any will add fragrance to the room and offer a pampering promise

A special way to enhance a bath with light fragrance is to find pre-packaged tub teas, which steep in warm bath water and provide a tonic for relaxation. Or you can fill a tea-straining ball with dried herbs and tea leaves and hang it under the faucet as the water runs.

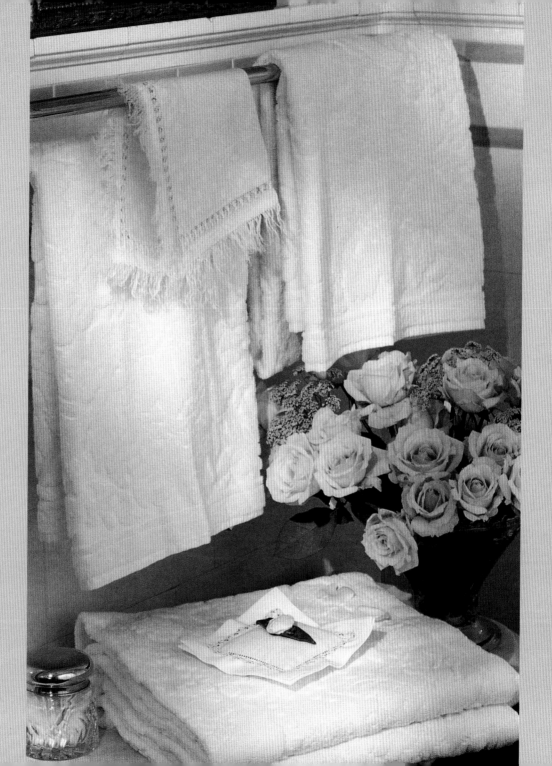

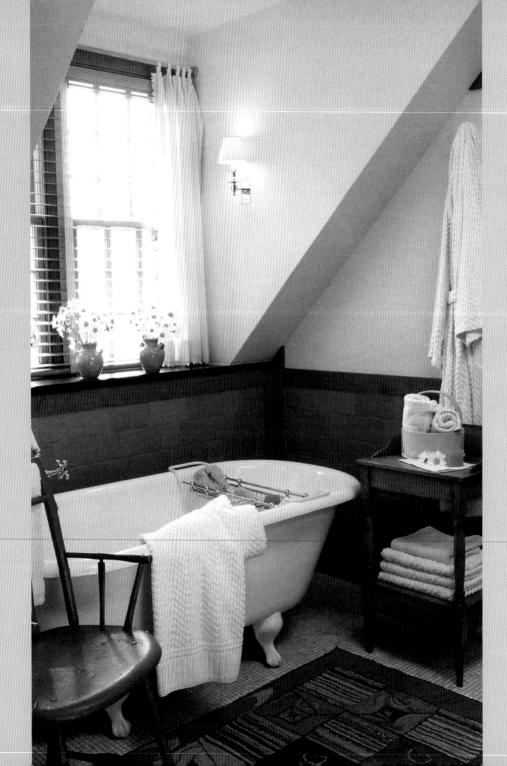

to guests. Roll up extra-large bath towels and place them in a large wicker basket with fragrant sachets, an offering as warm and comforting as an embrace. Add fresh flowers; even a single bloom in a clear vase speaks of a quiet welcome, a caring friend.

Think of your home as an exclusive inn that caters to the desires of your loved ones. Anticipate their needs and have available a few of the essentials of home: extra toothbrushes, a hotel-style bathrobe hanging on a hook, imported silkening soaps, powders, shampoos for different kinds of hair, lotions, and tools of beauty, such as a hair dryer, clear nail polish, a basket of cotton balls, and emery boards. Think of the guest bathroom as a chance to indulge yourself, too—you can buy in small quantities bottles of scents and lotions or aromatherapeutic bath oils that you might not otherwise try, or invest in just two expensive but irresistible towels, instead of an entire set. Put out beauty products in lovely containers, knowing that they will be appreciated by your guests.

If no spare bathroom exists to devote to guests, then prepare a small basket or brightly colored cosmetic bag with pampering goods, set out to greet them in whatever room will be their own.

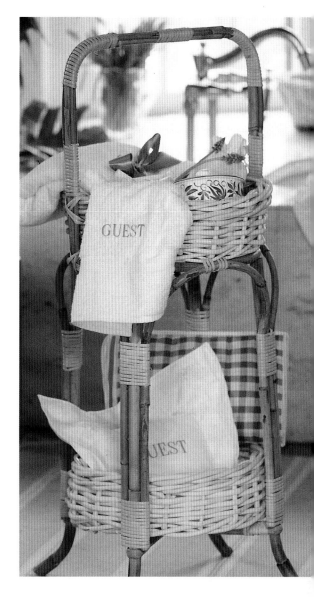

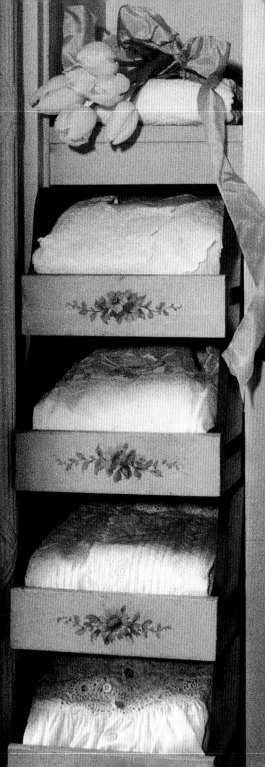

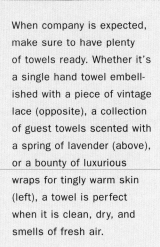

When company is expected, make sure to have plenty of towels ready. Whether it's a single hand towel embellished with a piece of vintage lace (opposite), a collection of guest towels scented with a spring of lavender (above), or a bounty of luxurious wraps for tingly warm skin (left), a towel is perfect when it is clean, dry, and smells of fresh air.

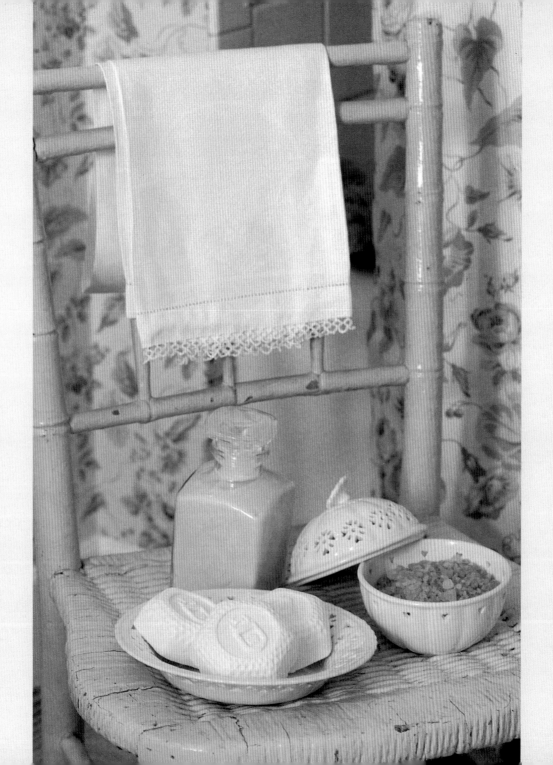

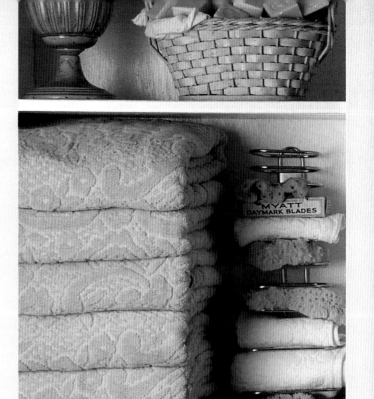

Cotton terry cloth, woven with a deep pile on one or both sides, is the most absorbent towel fabric. There are a variety of weaves and cotton yarns used in terry cloth for their decorative aspects or plain old softness. Chenille fibers are thick and have a soft but stubby feel when woven; combed cotton is more durable. Egyptian cotton, grown in the Nile Valley, is the most plush and produces long fibers, making for the softest, most absorbent towels. Dobby weaves incorporate flat, geometric figures into the larger picture, and is how bands are woven into towels; jacquards allow intricate designs to be woven on towels.

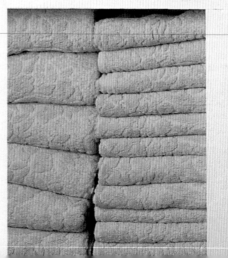

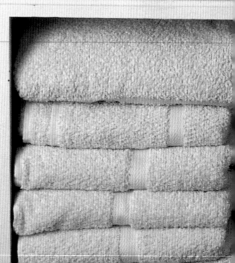

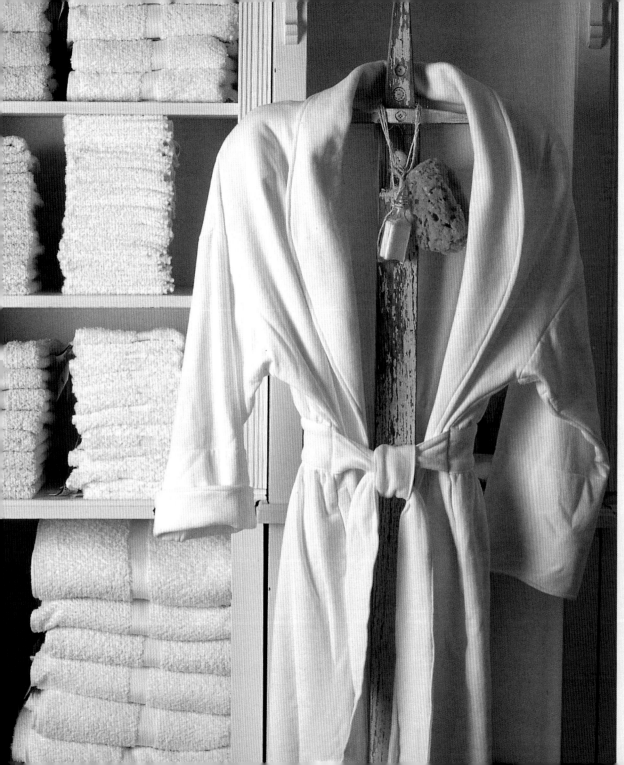

Fragrances to soothe the soul and arouse the spirits have been used since the beginning of time, when branches of juniper and cedarwood were burned in fires for their therapeutic aromas. In fact the word perfume comes from the words "par fume," meaning "by smoke." Today the warm resins of frankincense and myrrh and sweet sandalwood are burned to open the mind during meditation, help even breathing, and calm nerves.

Choosing a fragrance to wear isn't as easy as simply smelling something wonderful. Each person has a unique body chemistry that dictates the final scent of any perfume on skin, as well as how long it lasts. Don't select a fragrance at first whiff. The notes that encounter your nose first, called top notes, will dissipate quickly, within 30 seconds to three minutes. Top notes are built to lift your senses and induce you to buy the perfume. These notes will certainly compliment the final product, but will not last on the skin. The middle notes are a little richer, comprised of a blend of floral, fruity, green, spicy, or woody smells, and will last about ten minutes. The dry-down, or third layer of perfume, lasts for several hours. Before purchasing a perfume, spritz it on and see how it smells an hour later for a true sense of scent.

EVERY FRAGRANCE IS BASED ON A COMPLEX RECIPE OF NOTES

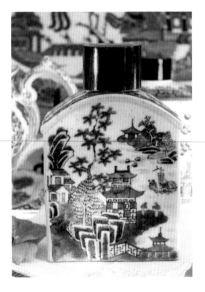

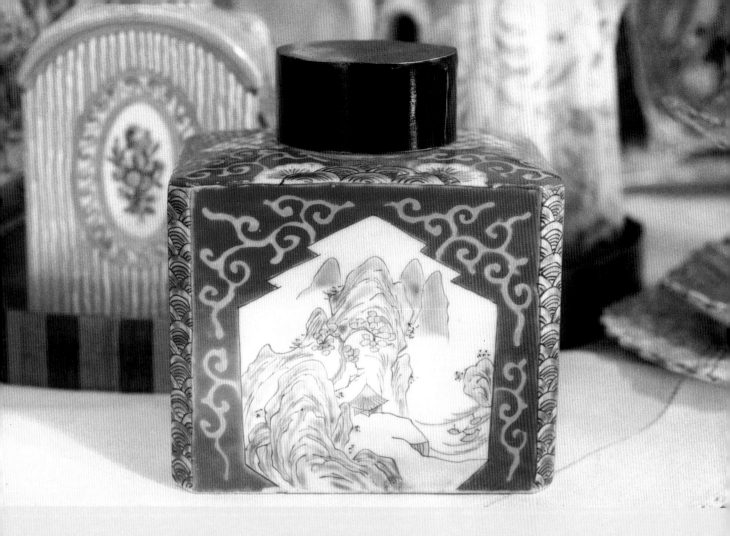

In this joyous holiday season, festive fragrances are used in potpourri under the mistletoe or worn out for the evening. Classic or new fragrances make a wonderful, feminine gift; antique perfume bottles or collectible toilet water flasks would make a treasured addition to any vanity table. Look at any jar, including an exquisite old tea caddie (above), as a possible container for lotions or small beauty items.

REST & REPOSE

By definition, beauty sleep is "extra" sleep, a midday nap after a full night's slumber. In our late lives, however, just getting to bed at a fair hour and sleeping through the night provides about as much beauty sleep as any of us get. In winter, our bodies want to hibernate, and sleep deprivation affects the quality of our work and life. It is also possible that our lack of dream-time may take a toll on our health. We do know that slumber is crucial for skin tone as well as sanity. Experts advise applying your most therapeutic treatments before bed, when they can work on the face uninterrupted for hours. Cosmetic chemists have even placed active ingredients like vitamin C in transdermal patches to be applied on wrinkles before bed time.

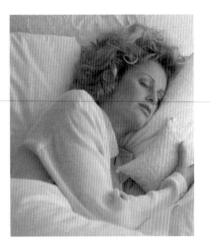

Scientists have found that when there is less than ten hours of daylight for a period of weeks, our bodies naturally fall into an apparently prehistoric state of sleep patterns, combining eight to nine hours a night of sleep with five or six hours of meditative wakefulness.

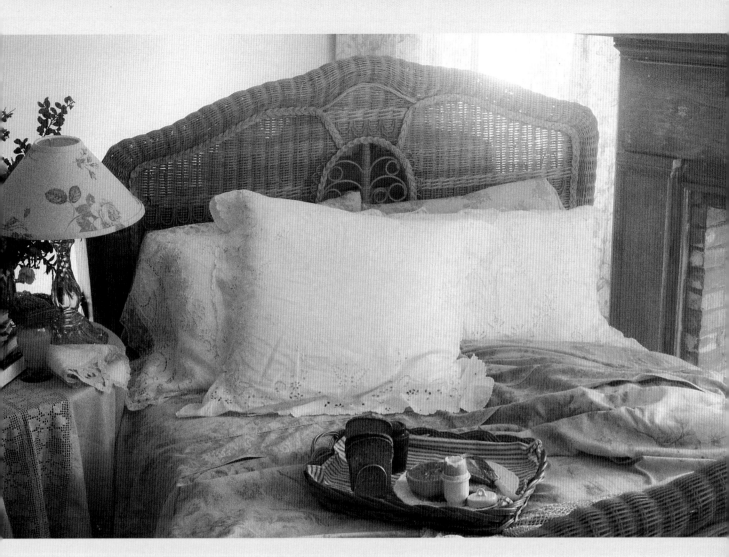

For the sweetest of dreams, create a scented pillow for your bed. Pack a small satin pillowcase with dried lavender, flaxseeds or rice, add a drop of lavender oil to enhance the fragrance, and sew it closed.

Place the dream pillow next to your head or gently over the eyes. The soft pressure against your eyes from the pillow and its sleep-inducing aroma will soon have you drifting into slumber.

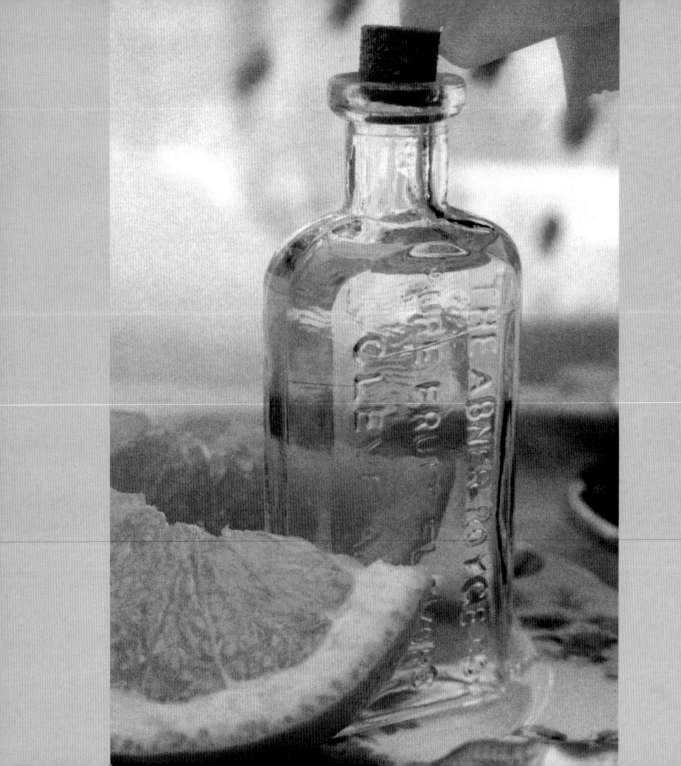

GIFT OF NATURE

Of all of winter's signature scents—pine, nutmeg, clove, gingerbread, cocoa—perhaps the most tantalizing are the tangy notes of tangerine, lemon, orange, and grapefruit. These tropical-toned fruits are especially refreshing when trees are bare and snow abounds. Slices of lemon, orange, and tangerine in a bath have mildly antiseptic properties, and their JUICE fresh, bright fragrance notes will wake up your senses. Neroli oil—obtained from orange blossoms and named for a princess who loved their odor—is also used as a fragrance in cosmetics and is considered to be anti-inflammatory, anti-bacterial and anti-fungal. Citrus is found in beauty products around the world. The Japanese use the unripe peels of a type of tangerine as a bath additive; the Chinese believe bitter Orange moves Chi, the body's energy; and Sri Lankans are known to drink lime juice to increase metabolism.

DRINK A CUP OF HOT WATER WITH THE OF A LEMON TO BALANCE THE SYSTEM

Essential oils of lemon, lime, and grapefruit are said to be anti-bacterial and are often used for their fragrances in soaps, creams, lotions, and perfumes.

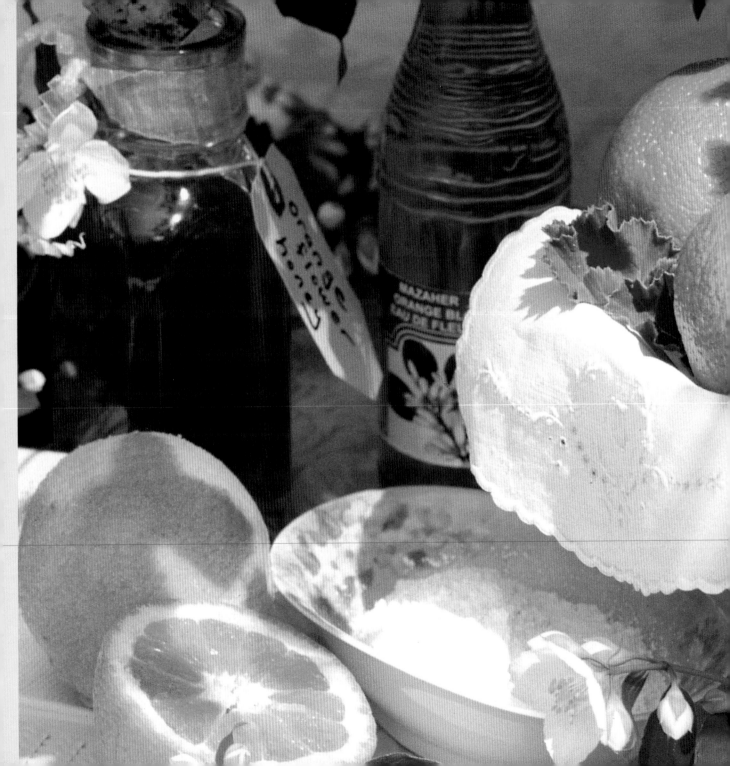

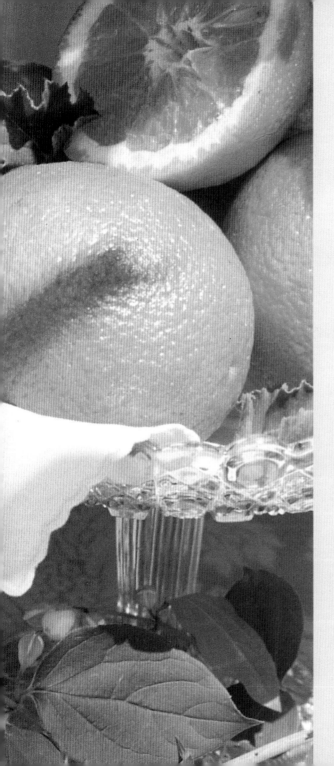

ORANGE-RIND FACIAL MASK

1 tbs. fresh-scented geranium leaves (lime geranium is especially nice)

2 tsp. freshly grated orange rind

1 1/2 tbs. orange flower water

1 tsp. orange flower honey

2 tsp. bentonite clay

Finely chop the geranium leaves in a coffee mill. Blend all the ingredients thoroughly and apply to your face in a slow, circular motion. Leave on for a few minutes, then rinse with tepid water and gently pat dry.

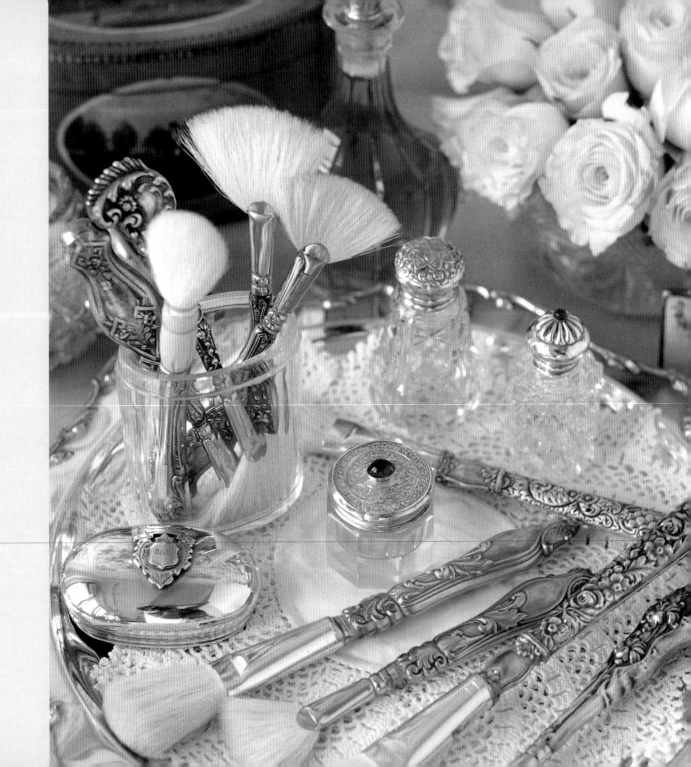

BEAUTY RITES
& RITUALS

During the winter, your body needs added care, in part because of the cold air outside and the recycled heat inside, both of which are drying to skin and hair. It is the time of year to moisturize, moisturize, moisturize. It is also the time of year when we overlook tending to ourselves in the midst of busily tending to everyone else.

One small thing to indulge in: makeup brushes. While they may seem superfluous (since most makeup comes with built-in applicators), for the most natural-looking makeup, invest in good brushes.

- Foundation brush: Small and flat, this brush is good for applying concealer or blending concealer with foundation.
- Eyeshadow brush: This allows more even and sheer coverage than a sponge-tip applicator, and makes it easy to wipe away mistakes or excess powder.

The best brushes are made with sable and have many silky bristles to hold makeup, are soft enough to apply makeup in one swoop, and are fluffy enough to easily blend makeup with your skin tone.

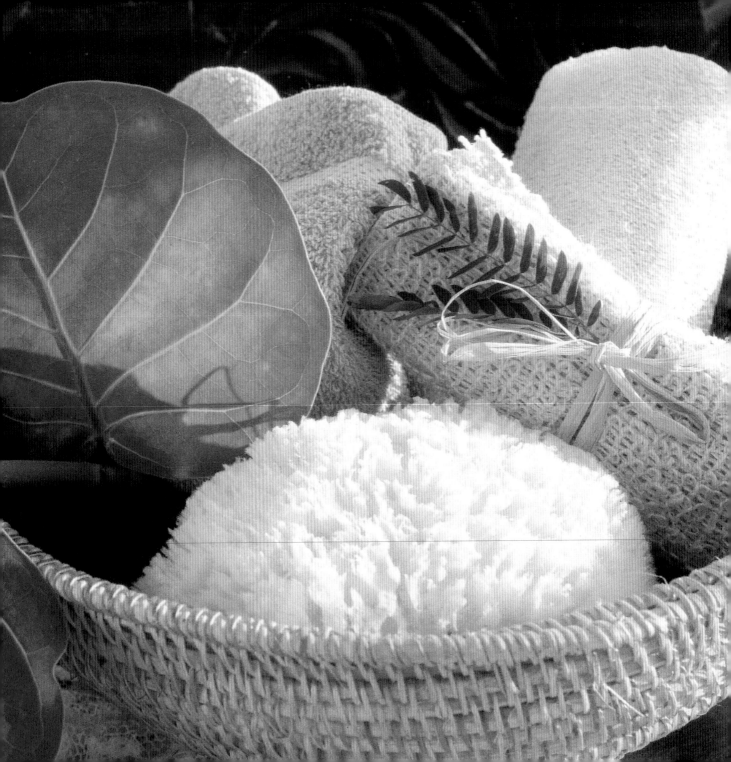

- Blush brush: Slightly smaller than a powder brush, this tool is crucial for blending blush so that it looks real. Move the brush in a circular motion, moving away from the nose.
- Powder brush: To use with loose powder; dip and tap off excess before applying. Also use this brush with pressed and bronzing powders.

Another of winter's indulgences is a leisurely soak. Place a vase of roses beside your tub, take a hot bath, then rinse in a cool shower to invigorate. Remember that each winter bath should have as its hidden agenda a hydrating effect on the skin. Elbows, knees, and heels may not be seen again until spring, but don't ignore them. Loofahs and sea sponges make gentle exfoliation an invigorating pleasure. Use a bath gel or liquid soap to create plenty of suds. Afterward, apply a rich moisturizer to still-damp skin, or try a soothing oil—perhaps coconut or sesame—to make skin glow.

DAILY RITUAL

Oft-overlooked feet need as much attention in the winter as they are due in the summer. Wrapped in socks and stockings, your feet hardly stand a chance at retaining moisture in this dry season. At the start and end of every day, rub the thickest cream or petroleum jelly onto your soles and toes to keep heels soft and cuticles manageable. Treat yourself to a bi-weekly pedicure, even if the thought of wearing sandals is as far off as a summer breeze.

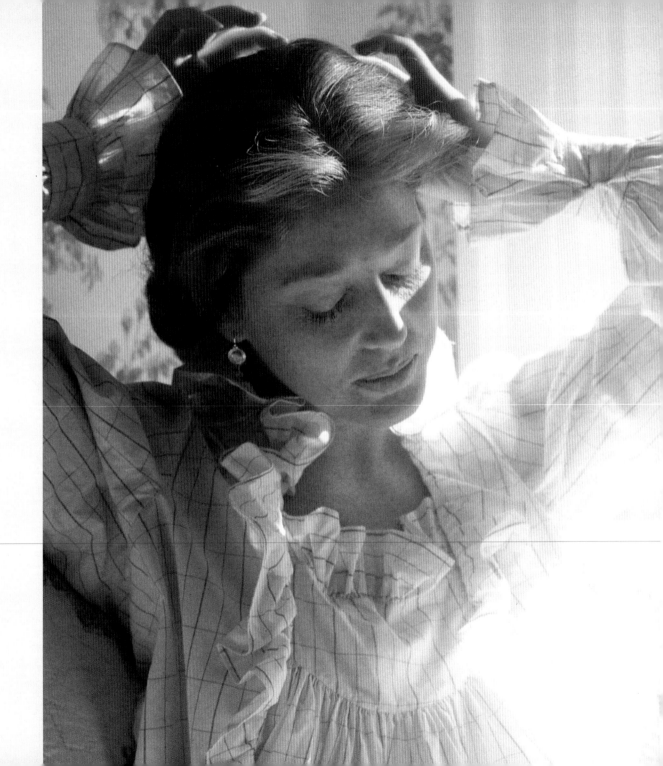

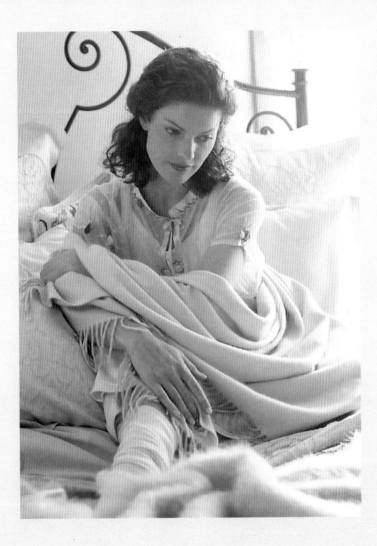

Winter Rituals

This is the season of extra-dry skin, washed-out faces, chapped lips, and fly-away hair. Here are a few ways to get through it:

- Change your skin care routine by selecting a creamier cleanser and a richer moisturizer than you use the rest of the year.
- If your face is flaking, avoid toners, which can be drying.
- For a quick makeup fix after you've been outside or to disguise dry skin: Add a dot of concealer over red blotches and blend well; follow with loose powder.
- To avoid hair static, spray the inside of your hat with hair spray; keep hair extra moist with a heavy conditioner or weekly hot oil treatment.
- Apply lip balm under or over lipstick to prevent chapping.

This the season to give gifts. A gift of makeup or luxurious skin cream will make a friend feel fabulous; products for lolling-in-the-tub will surprise a teacher or colleague. A single lipstick in a perfect shade or a lovely fragrance on its own make wonderful gifts, but consider creating gift baskets filled with an assortment of fine things. Choose a theme suited to the recipient. For a sailor or beachcomber, fill a large seashell with colored bath salts or bath beads, or put sunblock, lipbalm, and sunburn-soother in a wide-brimmed hat; a busy working mom would welcome relaxing bath oils, a recording of soft music, and a scented candle. For the gym-goer, create a basket of post-workout treats: a foot soak, invigorating shower gel, fluffy towel, and moisturizer. A teenage niece will like almost anything beauty-related: a collection of essential oils, or makeup brushes tied together with a bow and sprig of lavender.

CARING FOR TOOLS OF TOILETTE

Wash hairbrushes and combs regularly: mix 1 tablespoon of baking soda and 1/8 teaspoon of bleach or antiseptic cleanser in warm water. Soak 20 minutes, rinse and air dry. (Don't soak wooden or silver handles—just brush hair from the bristles and wipe the handles and bristle base with a damp, sudsy cloth.) Wash manicure tools in hot water after each use. Loofah sponges, which should be replaced every few months, can be washed in soap, hot water, and bleach. To wash makeup brushes, use a mild shampoo mixed with water, rinse well, and allow to air-dry. Another option is to pour a makeup dry cleaning solution on brushes and wipe off with a cotton cloth or tissue.

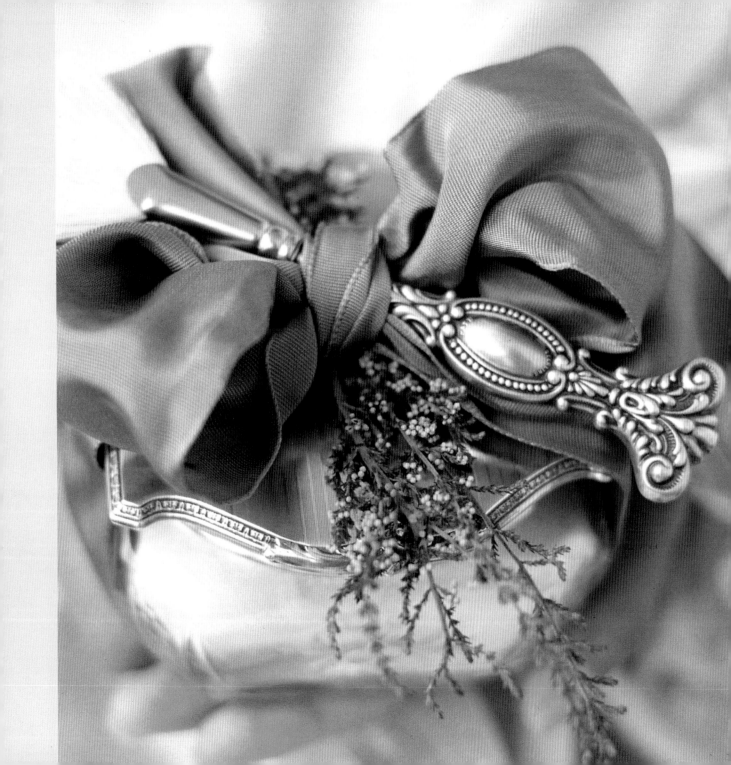

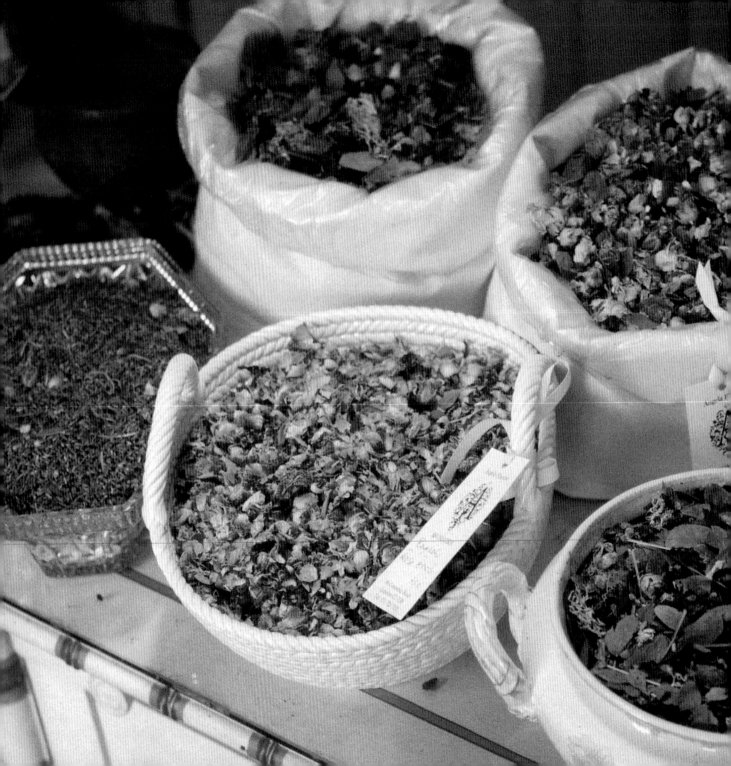

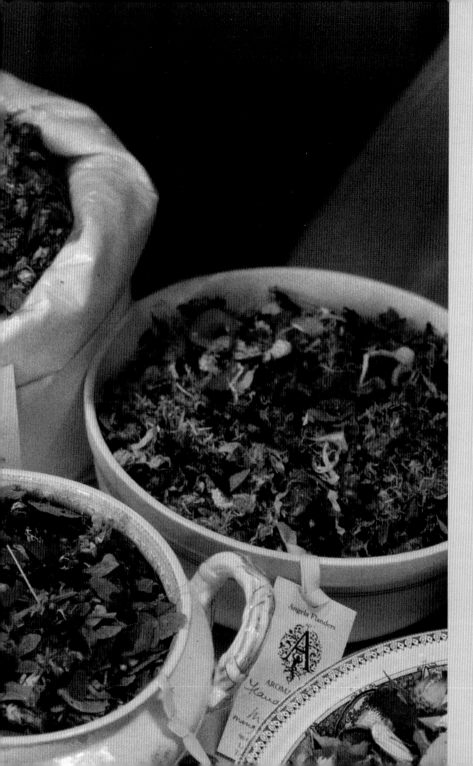

Because herbs have such wide beauty applications, grow as many as you can and dry them to use throughout the year, including them in handmade gifts at holiday time. The easiest way to dry herbs is to cut them early in the morning with sharp scissors (leave at least one-third of the plant behind so it will continue to thrive); tie stems in bunches no wider than one inch; and hang the bunches upside down. When completely dry—crisp to the touch—remove the buds and leaves and place them in air-tight containers. (To dry petals or citrus peels, spread them out on a screen or in a basket so air can circulate throughout, and gently stir from time to time until dry.)

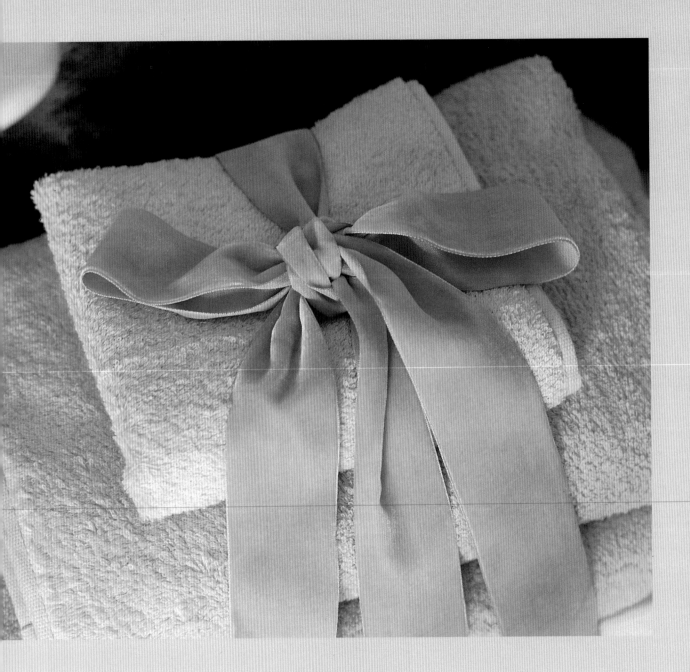

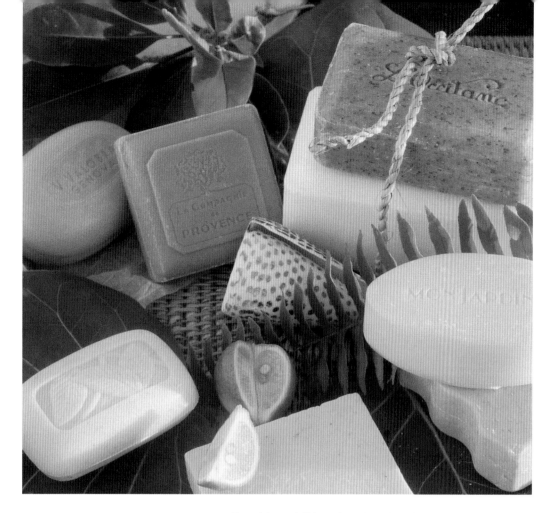

The widest of ribbons is like a kiss on plush towels (opposite), a gift for a newly married couple. For the person who doesn't like to admit to too fine a taste for luxuries, soaps in the most natural of tones (above) smell delicious enough to satisfy any appetite, and say "indulgence" without too much fuss.

Pleasure of *Scent*

Simple Hand and Body Lotion

2 ounces strong herb infusion

3/4 ounce lanolin or beeswax

3 ounces almond oil

To make an herb infusion, use the proportion of 4 to 6 tablespoons of a dried herb—or three times that amount of a fresh herb—to 1 cup of boiling water. Pour the water over the herbs, then let them steep until the water has cooled. Strain the tea through muslin or a coffee filter.

Melt the lanolin or the beeswax in the top of a glass or enamel double boiler. Gradually stir in the oil, beating continually with a wooden spoon. When the oil is incorporated, add the "tea" infusion in a thin stream, continuing to beat until blended. Remove from the heat and continue stirring until warm to the touch. Bottle and cap. As the lotion cools, shake occasionally.

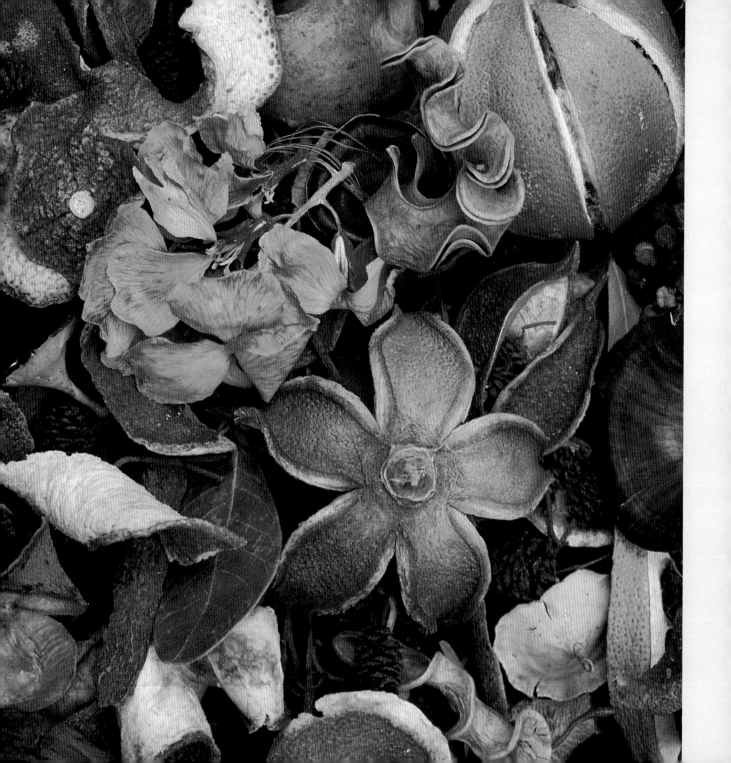

RESOURCES

Below is a list of suppliers and shops that offer unique and beautiful ingredients, products, and items for bath and beauty care.

AROMATHERAPY OILS, FLORAL WATER, AND SOAP

ANGEL'S EARTH
1633 Scheffer Avenue
St. Paul, MN 55116
(612) 698-3601
e-mail: a-earth@concentric.net
Essential oils

APHRODISIA
264 Bleecker Street
New York, NY 10014
(212) 989-6440
Essential oils, base oils, herbs, spices, natural soaps, bath salts, additive-free clay

CÔTÉ BASTIDE
The French Look, Inc.
363 West Erie Street
Chicago, IL 60610
(888) 690-8492
Soap, hair care, and bath products imported from France; call for store locations

CREATION HERBAL PRODUCTS
PO Box 344
10492 US Highway 421
Deep Gap, NC 28618
(704) 262-0006
http://www.creationherbal.com
Essential oils, herbs, glycerin, rose water, herbal extracts, infused oils

EAST END IMPORT COMPANY
PO Box 107
47 North Shore Road
Montauk, NY 11954
(516) 668-4158
Essential oils, floral water

LAVENDER LANE
7337 #1 Roseville Road
Sacramento, CA 95842
(916) 334-4400
www.choicemall.com/lavenderln/
donna@ricp.com
Essential and fragrance oils, lotions, gels, powders, books, kits, accessories, how-to recipes, bottles, jars

LORANN OILS
PO Box 22009
4518 Aurelius Road
Lansing, MI 48909
(800) 248-1302
Essential oils

NEFERTUM AROMATICS
45 Navy Street #A
Venice, CA 90291
(818) 754-0087 and
(800) 731-4950
Essential oils

SUGAR PLUM SUNDRIES
510 Notre Dame Avenue
Eastridge, TN 37412
(404) 297-0158
www.sugarplum.com
Handmade soap, essential oils

SUNFEATHER NATURAL SOAP CO.
1551 Route 72
Potsdam, NY 13676
(315) 265-3648
www.electroniccottage.com/
sunfeathersoaps/
Soap, essential oils, powdered clay, pumice

WOODSPIRITS HERB SHOP
1920 Apple Road
St. Paris, OH 43072
(937) 663-4327
Soap, salt scrubs, bath salts, powder, powder puffs, lavender and rose-geranium hydrosols

BEAUTY PRODUCTS

AROMA VERA
5901 Rodeo Road
Los Angeles, CA 90016-4312
(800) 669-9514
www.aromavera.com
Natural skin care and bath products, hair care, essential oils, books

AUBREY ORGANICS
4419 North Manhattan Avenue
Tampa, FL 33614
(800) 237-4270
**Natural skin, hair, and
bath products**

AVALON NATURAL COSMETICS
1105 Industrial Avenue
Petaluma, CA 94952
(707) 769-5120
**Natural cosmetics, hair care,
aromatherapy**

THE BODY SHOP BY MAIL
45 Horsehill Road
Hanover Technical Center
Cedar Knolls, NJ 07927
(800) 541-2535
**Bath and skin care
products, essential oils**

BODY TIME
1101 Eighth Street, Suite #100
Berkeley, CA 94710
(510) 524-0360
e-mail: btime@alink.net
**Bath and skin care products,
aromatherapy, essential oils**

CASWELL-MASSEY CATALOG
Catalog Division
100 Enterprise Place
Dover, DE 19901
(800) 326-0500
Bath, skin, and hair products

CRABTREE & EVELYN CATALOG
Mail Order Division
P.O. Box 158
Woodstock, CT 06281
(800) 272-2873
Bath and skin care products

ERBE AROMATHERAPY
196 Prince Street
New York, NY 10012
(212) 966-1445 and
(800) 432-ERBE
**Facial and skin care
products, essential oils**

KIEHL'S PHARMACY
109 Third Avenue
New York, NY 10003
(212) 475-4300
**Skin and hair care products,
essential oils**

POTPOURRI, TEAS, HERBS

AVENA BOTANICALS
219 Mill Street
Rockland, ME 04856
(207) 594-0694
**Herbs, herbal products,
teas, oils**

CHERCHEZ
P.O. Box 550
Millbrook, NY 12545
(800) 422-1744
**Dried flowers and herbs,
potpourri, room sprays**

FRONTIER COOPERATIVE
HERBS
Box 299
Norway, IA 53218
(800) 669-3275
**Herbs, spices, essential oils,
rose water, lavender water**

THE HERB SHOPPE
203 Azalea
Duenweg, MO 64841
(417) 782-0457
**Herbs, spices, botanicals,
oils, soaps, sundries**

HERBS, ETC.
1345 Cerrillos Road
Santa Fe, NM 87505
(505) 982-1265
Herbs, spices, floral water, dried flowers

MOUNTAIN ROSE HERBS
20818 High Street
North San Juan, CA 95960
(800) 879-3337
Herbs, teas, essential oils, herbal body care products, rose water, lavender water

NATURES' HERB COMPANY
1010 46th Street
Emeryville, CA 94608
(510) 601-0700
Herbs, spices, potpourri, oils

SAN FRANCISCO HERB COMPANY
250 Fourteenth Street
San Francisco, CA 94103
(800) 227-4530
www.sfherb.com
Dried herbs and flowers, essential oils

ST. JOHN'S HERB GARDEN
7711 Hillmeade Road
Bowie, MD 20720
(301) 262-5302
Herbs, essential oils, floral waters

A WORLD OF PLENTY
P.O. Box 1153
Hermantown, MN 55810-9724
(218) 729-6761
www.aworld@mindspring.com
Potpourri and sachet ingredients, fragrance oils, clays, powders

FRONTIER NATURAL PRODUCTS
Box 299
Norway, IA 52318
(800) 786-1388
www.frontiercoop.com
Organic dried herbs, bath and skin care products

BOTTLES, JARS, ACCESSORIES

SECOND CHANCE
45 Main Street
Southampton, NY 11968
(516) 283-2988
Vintage and antique glass bottles and apothecary jars

C.N. ART AND ANTIQUES
41 Union Square
New York, NY 10003
(212) 982-4985
Vintage and antique sterling-topped jars, bottles, and atomizers, hand-painted soap dishes, compacts, perfume bottles, sachets, sterling cosmetic brushes; by appointment

FACES OF TIME
32 West 40th Street, Suite 2D
New York, NY 10018
(212) 921-0822
Antique bottles, soap boxes, powder jars, small pitchers for bath oils

ZANGER COMPANY
7 Moody Road
Enfield, CT 06082
(800) 229-4687
Hand-painted ceramic soap and potpourri dishes, apothecary jars, bottles for lotions and oils

RECIPES & TREATMENTS

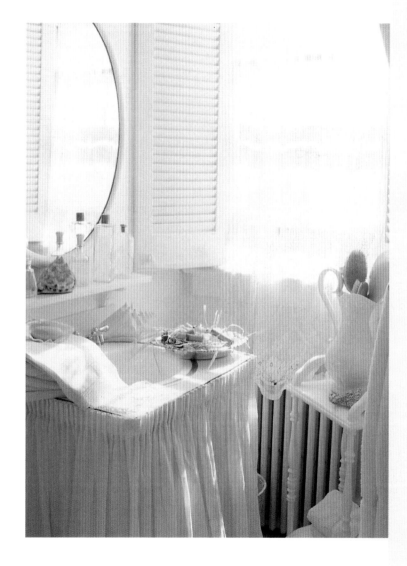

PHOTO CREDITS

2	Michael Skott	45	Luciana Pampalone	87	Thomas Hooper
4	Thomas Hooper	46	William P. Steele	89	Michael Skott
6	Toshi Otsuki	49	Luciana Pampalone	90	Toshi Otsuki
7	Michael Skott	51	Dominique Vorillon	91	Steven Randazzo
8	Luciana Pampalone	52	Tom Eckerle	92	Steven Randazzo
10	Luciana Pampalone	54	William P. Steele	95	William P. Steele (left),
12	Toshi Otsuki	56	Toshi Otsuki		Toshi Otsuki (right)
15	William P. Steele	57	Hedrich Blessing (left),	96	William P. Steele
16	Toshi Otsuki		Toshi Otsuki (right)	99	Luciana Pampalone
18	Toshi Otsuki	58	Luciana Pampalone	101	Tina Mucci
19	Jeff McNamara	61	Thomas Hooper	103	Toshi Otsuki
20	Luciana Pampalone	62	Toshi Otsuki	104	William P. Steele
22	Steven Randazzo	63	Thomas Hooper	105	Luciana Pampalone
23	Toshi Otsuki (left),	64	Luciana Pampalone	106	Toshi Otsuki (top),
	Pierre Chanteau (right)	66	Toshi Otsuki		William P. Steele (bottom)
24	Toshi Otsuki	68	Luciana Pampalone	107	Luciana Pampalone
27	Toshi Otsuki	70	Toshi Otsuki	108	Steven Randazzo
28	Michael Skott	71	Cynthia Warwick	109	William P. Steele
30	Sonia Bullaty	72	Wendi Schneider	110	Luciana Pampalone
32	William P. Steele	73	Toshi Otsuki	111	Thomas Hooper (left),
33	Pia Treyde	75	Jana Taylor		Toshi Otsuki (right)
34	Luciana Pampalone	76	Luciana Pampalone	112	Toshi Otsuki
35	Steven Randazzo	77	Luciana Pampalone	113	Toshi Otsuki (top),
36	Toshi Otsuki (left),	78	Toshi Otsuki		Steven Randazzo (bottom)
	Steven Randazzo (right)	80	Luciana Pampalone	114	Toshi Otsuki (top),
38	Toshi Otsuki	81	Toshi Otsuki		Jana Taylor (bottom)
40	Tina Mucci	83	Pia Treyde	115	Michael Skott
42	Jana Taylor	84	William P. Steele	117	Michael Skott

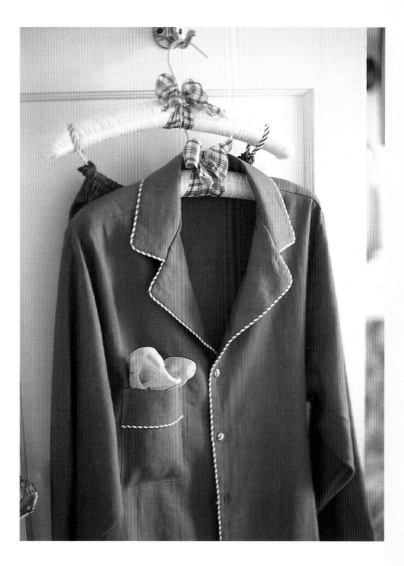

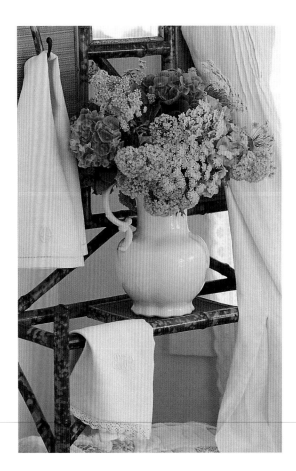